MEASUREMENT AND CLASSIFICATION OF PSYCHIATRIC SYMPTOMS

MEASUREMENT AND CLASSIFICATION OF PSYCHIATRIC SYMPTOMS

An Instruction Manual for the
PSE and Catego Program

J. K. WING
J. E. COOPER
N. SARTORIUS

CAMBRIDGE UNIVERSITY PRESS

Published by the Syndics of the Cambridge University Press
Bentley House, 200 Euston Road, London NW1 2DB
American Branch: 32 East 57th Street, New York, N.Y.10022

© Cambridge University Press 1974

Library of Congress Catalogue Card Number: 73-89008

ISBN: 0 521 20382 1
(ISBN of *Present State Examination* alone: 0 521 09850 5)

First published 1974

Printed in Great Britain
at the University Printing House, Cambridge
(Brooke Crutchley, University Printer)

CONTENTS

PREFACE

The good clinician, when he undertakes a diagnostic examination, knows what he
wants to find out. He makes a systematic exploration of the subject's mental state,
in order to discover whether any of a finite number of abnormal mental phenomena
are present. This manual is a guide to a particular method of standardising the
elements of this diagnostic process with a view to achieving comparability between
clinicians. The most important part of the book is therefore the glossary of definitions of symptoms. Everything else depends upon it. It is useless to try to determine
whether a symptom is present unless it is quite clear what its specific characteristics
are and how it can be distinguished from other symptoms. If the clinician knows
these differential definitions, the rest is a matter of technique. If he does not, no
amount of technical skill will give his judgements value.

The glossary of definitions is firmly grounded in the practice of the European
clinical school of psychiatry, with its long tradition of clinical observation and
emphasis on the importance of listening to the patient's description of unusual
experiences. The influence of this school has spread widely throughout the world
and we have found that most psychiatrists recognise that the procedures described
in this manual are a modification of their own practice. They are willing to adopt
the system for purposes of attaining comparability with colleagues, and the definitions of symptoms and the technical principles of interviewing are fairly simple to
learn and apply.

The only considerable exception we have found arises from the fact that an interview designed to discover whether defined symptoms are present must be based to
some extent upon the technique of 'cross-examination'. Patients find this completely acceptable and, to the extent that interviewer and patient are together
successful in producing an exact description of the symptoms, it can be a rewarding
and therapeutic experience in itself. However, members of some schools of
psychiatric thought, particularly the psychoanalytic, regard diagnosis as a relatively
unimportant part of their work and find cross-examination too 'directive' a method
of interviewing. This manual is not for them.

The PSE system has been developed over a period of ten years and it is still
evolving. It has been tested in a wide variety of settings. Various editions have been
translated and used in eleven languages apart from English, including Yoruba,
Hindi and Chinese, and thousands of patients have been interviewed with its help.

The latest edition is therefore based upon considerable experience but there is no doubt that it can be improved further. In particular, the method whereby data from the psychiatric history are taken into account, and the principles underlying the computer classification, Catego, are still in a relatively early stage of development. We shall welcome comments which will enable improvements to be incorporated in future editions, whether these are points of wording, suggestions about presentation, or modifications of rules of interviewing or classification. Above all we should welcome suggestions about defining symptoms more precisely or clearly. The system can be improved by dropping some of the symptoms, adding others, polishing the definitions of others and, in general, coming closer to the truth. There will certainly be a need for a further edition eventually.

1973

J. K. Wing
MRC Social Psychiatry Unit
Institute of Psychiatry
London

J. E. Cooper
Department of Psychiatry
University of Nottingham

N. Sartorius
Mental Health Unit
World Health Organisation

ACKNOWLEDGEMENTS

The PSE and Catego system have been evolving during a period of ten years and could not have reached the present level of development without the participation and advice of many colleagues. There have been three main groups of collaborators:

MRC SOCIAL PSYCHIATRY UNIT

The first six editions of the PSE were developed by the MRC Social Psychiatry Unit at the Institute of Psychiatry, London. The first paper was written by Professor J. K. Wing (Director of the Unit), Dr J. L. T. Birley, Dr J. E. Cooper, Dr P. Graham and Dr A. Isaacs. Clinical contributions were subsequently made by Dr Julian Leff and Dr Steven Hirsch. Statistical advice and assistance was given by Miss Pat Dugard, Miss Janice Nixon and Dr R. Hirschfeld. The programming was undertaken by Mrs Cynthia Taylor. Others who used various editions of the PSE, and whose data were helpful in development, were Dr A. O. Binitie, Dr J. Gleisner, Dr Sheila Mann, Dr P. Rohde and Dr Lorna Wing.

US–UK DIAGNOSTIC PROJECT

The principal investigator is Professor J. Zubin. Members of the New York team at the time of the investigations mentioned in this volume were Dr B. J. Gurland (Deputy Director), Dr L. Sharpe, Dr T. Farkas, Mr R. J. Simon, Miss P. Roberts and Miss V. Hoff. Members of the London team were Dr J. E. Cooper (Deputy Director), Dr R. E. Kendell, Dr J. R. M. Copeland, Dr N. Sartorius, Mrs A. J. Gourlay, Miss M. E. David, Miss Anne Vickery, Miss G. Stoneham and Mr B. S. Everitt.

WHO INTERNATIONAL PILOT STUDY OF SCHIZOPHRENIA

The collaborating investigators in this study have been:
 At Headquarters in WHO, Geneva; Dr N. Sartorius (principal investigator), Dr T.-Y. Lin (former principal investigator), Miss E. M. Brooke, Dr F. Engelsmann, Dr G. Ginsburg, Mr M. Kimura, Dr A. Richman and Dr R. Shapiro. In the field research centres in: Aarhus, Dr E. Stromgren (chief collaborating investigator), Dr A. Bertelsen, Dr M. Fischer, Dr C. Flach and Dr N. Juel-Nielsen; Agra, Dr K. C. Dube (chief collaborating investigator) and Dr B. S. Yadav; Cali, Dr C. Leon (chief collaborating investigator), Dr G. Calderon and Dr E. Zambrano; Ibadan, Dr T. A. Lambo (chief collaborating investigator) and Dr T. Asuni; London, Dr J. K. Wing

ix

(chief collaborating investigator), Dr J. Birley and Dr J. P. Leff; Moscow, Dr R. A. Nadzarov (chief collaborating investigator) and Dr N. M. Zharikov; Prague, Dr L. Hanzlicek (chief collaborating investigator) and Dr C. Skoda; Taipei, Dr C. C. Chen (chief collaborating investigator) and Dr M. Tsuang; Washington, Dr L. Wynne and Dr J. Strauss (chief collaborating investigators), Dr J. Bartko and Dr W. Carpenter.

A list of other staff contributing to the IPSS can be found in volume 1 of the Report of the IPSS, WHO, Geneva, 1973.

The part played by various individuals has been acknowledged at appropriate points in the text. The authors of this manual would like to record their deep appreciation of the fact that they have had the task of presenting work which has to a very considerable extent been based upon the collaborative efforts of a very large number of people, drawn from many professional disciplines.

1

MEASUREMENT AND CLASSIFICATION OF PSYCHIATRIC SYMPTOMS

1. WHY DESCRIBE OR CLASSIFY?

It is fashionable in some circles at the moment to decry the use of diagnostic labels, and to suggest that what doctors have to try to understand and treat are not diseases but problems, multifaceted and unclassifiable. A knowledge of the biological, psychological and social processes involved in problem-formation is recognised as indispensable, but to give some thought to their taxonomy is said to lead inevitably to sterile pigeon-holing, inflexibility and inhumanity. Giving a name to a condition, according to this view, not only serves little useful purpose but in the case of mental illnesses it can be positively harmful, since the label is often also a term of opprobrium or one implying hopelessness.

Doctors have done something to deserve these strictures by their unthinking use of disease terminology. People tend to be equated with cases; a unique individual becomes 'a leper' or 'a schizophrenic'. Doctors stand at the foot of the bed and discuss their patient, using an esoteric language which he is supposed not to understand. Medicine suffers from the disadvantages, as well as benefiting from the advantages, of being a well-established profession and institution. Its undoubted technical successes together with the age-old demand of patients to be treated and their accompanying willingness to believe well of those who treat them, must inevitably have dulled the self-criticism of the medical profession.

We begin with a statement of this point of view, not only because it represents a humane and continuing school of thought within medicine itself, but also because we wish to emphasise that nothing that we are going to say in this manual contradicts it. Above all in psychiatry, it is clear that people present with problems. Our primary aim is to make a contribution towards shaping and sharpening one of the tools needed by the doctor if he is to give more efficient help to people with psychiatric problems. If the medical practitioner confines himself to diagnosis and to treatment based specifically on it, the help he can give, though it may be of supreme importance in some special circumstances, is in general severely restricted. In fact, he himself becomes little more than an instrument and deserves an appropriate technical status. However, if the doctor cannot make a useful diagnosis he severely restricts his competence in a different way, and becomes immeasurably less useful to his patients.

Standing as we do at the vantage-point of half a century of achievement in scientific medicine, it is easy to see the relationship between groups of diseases that were once regarded as quite unconnected, and conversely we can see the necessity for breaking down other conditions once thought to be homogeneous into smaller subgroups by means of newly discovered criteria. Furthermore, in some important conditions, such as diabetes and hypertension, the processes underlying disease are now seen to be complex and even continuous, rather than discrete, as they were in some of the simpler and more obvious disease models provided, for example, by acute bacterial and viral infections.

In modern medicine and surgery, technical advances and laboratory aids to diagnosis are now so sophisticated that it is easy to slip into a way of thinking which tends to ignore the fact that all investigation and diagnosis still properly starts with interviewing the patient and making a provisional diagnosis on the basis of his past and present signs and symptoms. Psychiatry does not have sophisticated technical aids to diagnosis, but it must still lay a firm foundation of description and observation upon which future attempts to subdivide our present concepts will need to rest. A reasonable and careful concern with disease theories and systems of classification is appropriate for clinical psychiatry in its present state of development, and to neglect this stage would be to misunderstand the nature of scientific enquiry. Because we can now recognise that Tycho Brahe and Linnaeus were unduly preoccupied with description and with classification does not mean that astronomy and biology could have progressed without them. Kepler and Darwin built on the foundations laid by their predecessors. The same is true of pioneers such as Sydenham. Where would Claude Bernard and Virchow have been without forebears like him? Our present sophisticated medical knowledge has accrued because of centuries of observation and description, in which the describers and classifiers have played as dynamic and creative a part as those concerned with process. It is hardly helpful to tell psychiatrists that there is no need to begin at the beginning; that Kraepelin was unnecessary and that all they have to do is to look at their patients' problems. Such advice, if taken seriously, is likely to be translated into a purely *ad hoc*, symptomatic approach, or one in which any theory is acceptable since none is meant to be tested.

At the very least, therefore, psychiatric disease theories need to be given a fair test. Such a conclusion is fully compatible with the assumption that other types of observation and other types of theory may also usefully be applied to help patients. Doctors are not only diagnosticians; they are teachers, psychologists, social workers and pastoral counsellors. Theirs is a highly complex role, but it is one which cannot properly be carried out without specialised tools. Diagnosis is such a tool. There is no doubt that disease theories have been of immense value in the development of many fields of medicine and in practical application to help patients. What we have to discover is how far they are useful in psychiatry.

There are two parts to such an investigation. In the first place, we need to know whether there are clinically recognisable syndromes which all psychiatrists can agree upon and label in the same way. If this demonstration is successful, in the case of a given clinical syndrome, it does not mean that a disease theory applies, merely that a disease theory can be tested. However, the value of this first step should not be underestimated. Early childhood autism may be taken by way of example. In 1799, at the time of the French Revolution, Itard wrote a treatise describing the symptoms and the treatment of a boy, discovered in the woods near Aveyron, who would now be called autistic. Itard anticipated practically all the developments of recent years (Itard, 1932). He was a forerunner of Montessori and he had enormous influence on the way diagnosis, treatment and services developed. His description of early childhood autism is easily recognisable today. But he did not realise that he was dealing with a distinct syndrome. The wild boy of Aveyron, to Itard, was either a unique example of lack of education or he was an idiot. It was not until Kanner (1943) recognised, isolated and described the syndrome that real advance could be made. Itard's insights could then be applied to other children with the same condition. Kanner's first step was of incalculable value. No disease theory can be elaborated before the clinical syndrome has been recognised and labelled. The second step can then be taken, which is to test the validity of various explanatory theories.

This book is mainly devoted to two questions connected with the first step. First, whether certain psychological and behavioural phenomena which have generally been thought by psychiatrists to be 'symptoms' of mental illnesses can be reliably recognised and described, irrespective of the language and culture of the doctor or patient; secondly, whether rules of classification can be specified with such precision that an individual with a given pattern of symptoms will always be allocated to the same clinical grouping. If these two conditions could be fulfilled we should be in a position to proceed to the second stage of investigation, that is, to test individual disease theories. We can do nothing, however, if the first stage proves unsuccessful.

2. THE CONCEPT OF ILLNESS

The literal meaning of 'pathology' is the science of disease. Most well-developed disease theories are based upon a knowledge of the homeostatic mechanisms which maintain some relevant bodily function such as blood sugar within known limits. When certain causal factors operate, the normal cycle is upset, the limits are exceeded, and a clinical syndrome such as diabetes mellitus becomes manifest. Thus the disease theory is derived from a theory of normal biological functioning.

The clinical syndrome may, of course, present in purely psychological terms even though it is physically based. An experience of pain in the centre of the chest radiating down the left arm is characteristic of ischaemic heart disease. Edwards (1971) points out that pain a few seconds after swallowing solid food is a highly discriminating symptom; the diagnosis (oesophageal stricture) is virtually contained in this description. Other manifestations of the pathophysiology can be seen in behaviour or observed by special techniques of examination. Diagnosis is less often made than it used to be on the basis of the patient's subjective account alone, but the 'history' is still the main foundation of medical consultation.

In psychiatric practice there is often nothing else to go on but the patient's own description of his experiences. However, since doctors have been making examinations of 'mental state' from time immemorial, they do not have to start afresh each time but can utilise the experience of their predecessors. Certain clinical conditions are recognised by most psychiatrists all over the world as 'syndromes', that is, clusters of traits which frequently occur together at one point in time, or which follow a characteristic sequence over a number of months or years. If we exclude conditions such as dementia, delirium or severe mental retardation, in which a structural lesion is frequently evident, the psychological syndromes most generally thought important are those of anxiety, depression, obsession, hysteria and various types of delusion and/or hallucination. In each case, it would generally be agreed that there are groups of syndromes, rather than one unitary state, so that no single disease theory is likely to apply. In many cases, there are also observable bodily abnormalities; most evident in the case of anxiety states, least evident perhaps in obsessional conditions, but nowhere sufficient in themselves for a reliable classification.

Clinicians are by no means unanimous that even these broad syndromes can be reliably recognised, but there is a sufficient degree of agreement to make the possibility worth investigating. As to the explanation of why the syndromes occur, many schools of thought have proliferated. The central one uses the analogy of biological disease. It is postulated that underlying each clinical syndrome there is some normal biological mechanism, perhaps neurophysiological or neurochemical in nature, which has gone wrong through the operation of complex causes. As with better understood disease models, some of the contributing causes can be psychological or social as well as biological. It is well accepted that there may be links between the syndromes and that the syndromes themselves may be far from unitary; for instance, the parallels between a disease theory of schizophrenia and a disease theory of diabetes mellitus are immediate and striking (Wing, 1974). The disease model of any functional psychiatric syndrome is most obviously deficient, however, at the point where evidence is most needed; that is, at the point where a link has to be made between the psychological characteristics which clinicians recognise as a syndrome and the underlying hypothetical biological process. This is true of all the major functional psychiatric syndromes and is the reason why they are called 'functional'. Evidence that there is such a link is only indirect, examples being: a raised incidence in relatives not obviously explicable in environmental terms, the occurrence of biological precipitating factors (e.g. schizophrenic symptoms occurring after amphetamine intoxication), the involvement of the little-understood biological mechanisms underlying attention and communication, the response to specific forms of medication and the development of typical patterns of chronic impairments.

There is enough evidence here to suggest that psychiatric disease theories can be useful in everyday clinical practice. At the very least, a strong case can be made that they ought to be more systematically and comprehensively tested. This requires a more precise use of terminology than is currently practicable, since there is good evidence that terms like 'schizophrenia' and 'affective disorder' are used very differently in different parts of the world.

The difficulties lying in the way of reaching agreement on terminology are discussed in the following two sections of this chapter. Basically, a psychiatrist collects three kinds of information in order to make a diagnosis: a 'present state' description, which may be repeated several times, the purpose of which is to evaluate the morbid phenomena experienced by the patient and any evidence of abnormality in behaviour; a clinical history, which indicates what symptoms have occurred during previous episodes of illness; and other information concerning possible causes or pathology, e.g. laboratory data or response to a specific treatment. A set of classifying rules is more or less consciously applied to this material in order to arrive at a diagnostic class. Most of the information is derived from the interview and any attempt at standardisation must therefore begin at this stage.

3. DESCRIPTION OF PSYCHIATRIC SYMPTOMS*

In deciding which symptoms are present at any particular point in time, the psychiatrist is influenced by three major factors; his method of interview, his definition of symptoms and the responses of the patient. Each of these components can vary independently of the others but they are also to some extent interdependent. The least standardised method is to use a self-rated questionnaire. The commonest technique of standardisation is to use a checklist of items, each more or less defined in clinical terms, without any attempt at standardising the form of the examination. Such systems have been reported by Foulds (1965), Lorr et al. (1963), Overall and Gorham (1962) and Wittenborn (1955). Lists of items useful for describing depression have been published by Hamilton (1960) and Beck et al. (1961) and for anxiety by Taylor (1953). The use of such lists reduces variability to some extent and under some circumstances reliability can be high. However, the examiner's symptom definitions, the threshold at which he judges a symptom to be present, his techniques of eliciting symptoms and of dealing with different interviewing conditions and different responses from patients, are not brought under control.

A much more closely standardised psychiatric interview has been described by Spitzer and his colleagues (1964, 1967, 1970). The questions to be asked by the examiner are laid down and instructions on how to code the answers are included in the schedule. The symptoms to be rated are not, however, defined in any detail. Reliability is on the whole satisfactory. In the latest version, which is based upon

* The term 'symptom' will be used throughout as shorthand for 'symptom of a hypothetical underlying disease process' but its significance would not be altered if some more neutral term, such as 'trait', were substituted.

factor analysis of data collected using the previous versions (Endicott and Spitzer, 1972) nineteen scales are rated, only twelve of them symptomatic, including one rating for anxiety, one for depression, and one for all varieties of hallucinations. The selection of items and the relative lack of interest in the details of psychopathology, particularly in those that might be of diagnostic importance, is American rather than European in style.

In contrast, the 'AMP-system' (Scharfetter, 1971) contains a much more detailed checklist of items, each with a brief definition, which includes symptoms such as thought broadcast, thought withdrawal, thought insertion, delusions of outside influence, etc., which the American list omits. Training courses were organised and videotaped and filmed interviews used to instruct users. There is, however, no schedule for guiding the conduct of the interview.

The work described in this present volume goes further than any of these other attempts to standardise psychiatric procedures, with the final aim of making the eventual choice of a diagnostic term more reliable. The two major components of the process by which a symptom is accepted or rejected are brought under control; these are, first, the interviewing technique by which the patient's complaints are elicited, and second, the use of an agreed set of descriptions or definitions of the symptoms in question. In addition, a system is made available by which the condensation of symptoms with syndromes and finally into diagnoses can be made by unvarying criteria.

This work started with the development of a comprehensive list of questions, with brief symptom definitions, and a detailed guide to the conduct of the interview, published after five years of development by Wing and his colleagues (1967). This 'Present State Examination' (PSE) is based on the common medical interview technique of cross-examination. The clinician has in mind a particular symptom and, in order to be sure whether the patient has it or not, asks a series of questions, each one depending on the patient's previous reply. Only if he is satisfied that the symptom is indeed present is a positive rating made. The patient's affirmation is not in itself sufficient. The criteria laid down for the presence or absence of a symptom are fairly detailed. The symptom of worrying, for example, is only rated if the patient says that he has a round of painful thought, out of proportion to the subject of the worry, which he cannot voluntarily stop. This is a very flexible method which allows the examiner liberty to vary the procedure in response to different interviewing conditions or patients' reactions while still pursuing an agreed goal. It requires expert clinicians. Reliability was studied in detail, both by comparing several clinicians rating one interview and by comparing different interviewers rating the same patient at an interval of a few days. In general, it was satisfactory (see chapter 5).

In summary, these methods indicate that it is possible to rate the presence or absence of a wide range of psychiatric symptoms reliably through the use of special techniques, and this fact suggests that part, at least, of the variability in making psychiatric diagnoses can also be reduced.

4. THE CLASSIFICATION OF SYMPTOMS

The term classification may be used in two ways, to mean the system of classes into which objects or data are sorted and also the process of allocation of each object to a class. Hempel (1959) suggests that the ideal classification should be mutually exclusive and jointly exhaustive; that is, each object should be allocated to one class and to one class only, and a class should be available for each object, thus ensuring a minimum of uncertainty and ambiguity.

There are many possible techniques for classifying abnormal mental states but the most familiar is clinical diagnosis. Here the psychiatrist follows a set of rules which he has previously learned and modified in the light of his own experience to the clinical information he collects about his patients. Foulds (1965), who reviewed the evidence concerning the reliability with which psychiatrists classified psychiatric conditions, suggested that there was very little evidence in the few, mostly inadequately-conducted studies then published, to justify a wholesale condemnation such as that made by Roe (1949). Foulds based this judgement on the fact that the main outlines of the classical Kraepelinian scheme tended to persist in spite of criticism (the implication being that no one could suggest anything better), that classifications derived by factor analytic means (e.g. Wittenborn, 1951; Lorr, Klett, McNair and Lasky, 1963; Lorr, 1965, 1966) tended to look very like clinical diagnoses and that various studies had shown that broad diagnostic categories could be fairly reliably allocated by clinicians working in everyday practice (Schmidt and Fonda, 1956; Kreitman, 1961). There is, of course, general agreement that current nosology needs to be greatly improved.

One technique suggested as an alternative is based on factor analysis or cluster analysis of material derived from the check lists described earlier. Lorr, for example, applied factor analytic techniques to ratings on the IMPS, producing empirical groupings such as 'perceptual distortion' or 'paranoid projection'. Such statistical categories are, of course, even less validated than clinical diagnoses but they have the merit of being derived according to a fully specifiable procedure in which there are no elements of subjective judgement, once the ratings of IMPS items have been made. It is understandable that most of these systems have been produced in the United States since, as Lorr (1966) pointed out, 'in much of American psychiatry, formal diagnosis is actually ignored as relatively unimportant and outmoded, or disparaged as nondynamic and useless'.

Fleiss, Gurland and Cooper (1971) carried out a factor analysis of the data collected in the US–UK Diagnostic Project (Cooper et al., 1972), which were derived from a combined schedule incorporating both the items in the PSE schedule (Wing et al., 1967) and those in the PSS schedule developed by Spitzer and his colleagues (Spitzer et al., 1970). It was demonstrated that phobic anxiety could be factorially separated from depression, flat affect from retarded speech and retarded movement, and observed restlessness from mania. These distinctions would be expected on

clinical grounds by clinicians who regard such matters as important, but they could not have been made unless the relevant items had been included in the PSE schedule. PSE data from the US–UK Project were also used in a cluster analysis by Everitt, Gourlay and Kendell (1971), who showed that two different cluster techniques produced groups identifiable with manic and depressive phases of manic-depressive disorders, with paranoid schizophrenia and with residual schizophrenia. Thus it is clear that the output of factor and cluster analytic studies depends very much upon the input. It is impossible to obtain certain clusters from PSS or IMPS data, simply because the relevant items have not been included.

Spitzer and Endicott (1968, 1969) have employed another classification technique, that of a set of clinical rules embodied in a computer program, DIAGNO II, using as input the ratings on current and past psychopathology obtained from the standardised interview, CAPPS (Endicott and Spitzer, 1973). The agreement with clinical diagnosis was rather low, but it was as high as the agreement between clinicians. Fleiss *et al.* (1973) compared three methods for generating psychiatrists' diagnoses, all based on CAPPS ratings: Bayes, discriminant function and DIAGNO II. The third technique performed best on a cross-validation sample drawn from a new population but the agreement with clinical diagnosis remained rather low.

The development of a similar set of diagnostic rules (Wing, 1970, 1971), based on European clinical practice, and using PSE data as input, is described in chapter 6, and its relationship to the clinical diagnoses used in two large international studies is discussed in chapter 7.

5. OTHER DATA RELEVANT TO THE DIAGNOSIS

Data from previous episodes of illness may have relevance to the current diagnosis but there has been little attempt at systematic study. Simon *et al.* (1971) examined the effect on diagnosis of a lengthy interview concerning the development of illness. There were changes in major diagnostic category in only 15% of cases when the historical information was made available, compared to PSE information only. Most of these changes occurred when there was uncertainty in the diagnosis. Sartorius, Brooke and Lin (1970) described a diagnostic exercise which also suggested that 'present state' information was more important than historical diagnosis. It must, however, be remembered that the PSE covers the last month, and so is by no means a description at a point in time; in addition, patients very often refer to their previous illnesses and symptoms when describing the recent ones, so it is common for the interviewer to be presented with a complicated mixture of information, relating to the present, the recent past and the remote past, which, even though the ratings are made so far as possible on what has occurred during one month, makes an absolute comparison of the effects of 'present state' with 'historical' information difficult. Further information on the addition of historical data will be found in chapters 4 and 7.

The value of standardising the addition of aetiological information has yet to be investigated.

6. PLAN OF THIS BOOK

There are several components in the PSE–Catego system, some of which can be used independently of the others. They may be listed as follows:

1. The PSE interview and glossary of definitions of symptoms, which may be used on its own as a standardisation of the diagnostic examination common in European and much world psychiatry.

2. The PSE check list of symptoms, each of which can be rated as absent or present in moderate or severe form.

3. The syndrome check list (SCL) which can conveniently be used to rate episodes of psychiatric illness if the information available is not sufficiently detailed to rate symptoms.

4. The Catego computer program, which incorporates a set of clinical diagnostic rules designed to classify PSE or SCL data into descriptive classes which (when data from the aetiology schedule have been added, or organic causes excluded) can be compared with grouped rubrics from the International Classification of Diseases.

It would be quite possible to use the PSE interview for clinical or teaching purposes without making the ratings. It is virtually a miniature text book of 'functional' psychopathology. Similarly the symptom list or the syndrome check list can be used on their own to give descriptive profiles, and to measure change. The various components are described separately.

Chapter 2 describes the development of the PSE through several editions and sets out the general principles underlying its administration. Chapter 3 shows how the 500–600 items in the seventh and eighth editions were condensed to yield the 140 symptoms which are directly rated in the ninth and latest edition, and for which a glossary of differential definitions is provided. Chapter 4 describes the further condensation necessary to reduce 140 symptoms to 38 syndromes, which can be directly rated in the syndrome check list. All versions of the PSE become comparable at the syndrome stage. Chapter 5 discusses the reliability of measurement of item, symptom, syndrome and diagnosis based upon the PSE interview. Chapter 6 contains details of the Catego computer program which incorporates a system of diagnostic rules acting on PSE or SCL ratings in order to allocate each condition finally to one descriptive class, thus simulating the processes of clinical diagnosis. The results obtained in two large international studies are used to illustrate these techniques in chapter 7. Chapter 8 contains a discussion of the uses of the PSE and Catego system in the light of the problems already discussed above.

2

DEVELOPMENT AND
ADMINISTRATION OF THE PSE

1. MAIN PURPOSES OF THE PSE

The Present State Examination (PSE) schedule is a guide to structuring a clinical interview, with the object of assessing the 'present mental state' of adult patients suffering from one of the neuroses or functional psychoses. The PSE was developed in order to provide reliable and precise data concerning the patient's clinical condition which, in spite of being expressed in numerical form, would still remain intelligible to the clinician and usable by him. This ideal can never be completely attainable because of the difficulties of defining and measuring such complex and often abstract concepts and phenomena, but it has always been kept in mind. Whenever there has been any conflict between clinical and statistical judgement, clinical judgement has been allowed to prevail.

The data collected in this way are intended to serve three main purposes:

(i) To provide a reliable method of examining the 'present mental state' of an individual at a given point in time and of describing which symptoms and syndromes are present. This aim is basically descriptive. Symptom and syndrome profiles can be used for comparative purposes, to measure change, and for matching and selection. If a standard set of classifying rules could be developed, the symptom ratings could also be used to allocate each individual to a descriptive class. This aim was the most important one in determining the characteristics of the interview.

(ii) To allow the investigation of diagnostic rules and practices. A reliable system of measurement and classification allows a comparison between the diagnosis given by clinicians and the class allocated by the standard procedure. A consideration of the degree of concordance and type of discrepancy between the two classifications should throw light on the processes of clinical diagnosis and suggest how they might be improved. At best, new light might be thrown on the nature of the conditions themselves.

(iii) To provide a clear-cut basis for teaching and clinical work. This is the least of the aims, since the PSE was developed as a research instrument. If the other two aims were achieved, however, it would be expected that there would be educational and clinical uses as well.

2. DEVELOPMENT OF THE PSE

The items in the PSE schedule were originally chosen by a small number of physicians to represent their current clinical practice and teaching. Subsequent changes have been made in the same way. Increasing experience as more and more psychiatrists became involved has led to many changes, but the basic clinical viewpoint has not fundamentally altered. Indeed, it has become clear that the PSE incorporates the views of a school of thought which might reasonably be called Western European in its origins and which is shared by psychiatrists in many·other parts of the world.

The development of the first five editions is described in an article by Wing *et al.* (1967). Since then further development has taken place in the light of experience of its use in several large international projects and many smaller and more intensive studies. The latest edition is the ninth and this is the one which is presented in full in the present manual. Most of the available statistical data, however, are derived from the seventh and eighth editions, and there are several versions of each of these. A brief note is therefore appended, describing each of the main versions of the schedule.

SEVENTH EDITION

The seventh edition was produced by the original authors in the light of experience with the earlier versions and of suggestions from T. Y. Lin (then of WHO), E. Strömgren (Aarhus) and L. Wynne (Bethesda). It was used by the US–UK Diagnostic Project, in their Netherne and Brooklyn studies; the 'combined schedule' incorporated many items from Spitzer's Mental Status Schedule as well, in order to compare the two. The numbering of items was therefore different to that in the version used by the MRC Social Psychiatry Unit, but the items themselves were identical. Work in which the seventh edition was used has been published from the US–UK project (Kendell *et al.*, 1968; Cooper *et al.*, 1972) and the MRC Social Psychiatry Unit (Brown, Birley and Wing, 1972). The schedule was also used in the preliminary phase of the WHO International Pilot Study of Schizophrenia (WHO, 1973). A set of instruction manuals was produced for the seventh edition, together with illustrative audio-tapes and video-tapes. These are superseded by the present manual.

EIGHTH EDITION

The eighth edition is an expanded version of the seventh, with a modified scoring system and many extra items, about 500 in all. Suggestions from the collaborators in the IPSS and the US–UK Diagnostic Project and from Dr Felix Post (London) were incorporated. There are three main versions.

The MRC eighth edition will be the one used for purposes of illustration in subsequent chapters. Copies are available to those interested in the development of the PSE but, for reasons of economy of space, it is not printed in this manual. Publications referring to its use in MRC projects are by Hirsch and Leff (1971), Leff and Wing (1971) and L. Wing *et al.* (1972). It has also been used by Binitie (1971) in Benin, Nigeria.

The US–UK eighth edition is identical to the MRC version but was used in the form of a combined schedule that incorporated Spitzer's Mental Status Schedule so that the numbering of items is different. Its use is described by Cooper *et al.* (1972).

The WHO eighth edition is a shortened version containing only 360 items, concentrating mainly on the psychotic symptoms, specially modified to suit the requirements of the IPSS. The collaborating investigators translated the schedule into the languages of the study. It is described by Sartorius, Brooke and Lin (1970) and in the first volume of the IPSS report (WHO, 1973). Copies are available from the Mental Health Unit, WHO.

NINTH EDITION

The ninth edition is the latest and is based upon all the experience gained in the earlier studies. During the analysis of data from the seventh and eighth editions it became clear that most of the phenomena likely to be encountered during a present state examination can be covered by rating the presence or absence of 140 symptoms, and the main change in the ninth edition is this reduction. However, most of the original questions have been retained, although a two-tier system of questioning has been introduced (analogous to an extra cut-off system) so that the obligatory questions have been markedly reduced in number. The rating of severity of each symptom is also made more uniform and the schedule is, in general, easier to use and takes a shorter time to administer. Details are given in chapter 3.

Early drafts of the ninth edition have been used in studies which have since been published (Leff and Vaughn, 1972; Gleisner, Hewett and Mann, 1972; Hirsch *et al.*, 1973; Mann and Sproule, 1972). Valuable suggestions from R. Gaind, S. Hirsch, J. Leff and P. Rhode have been incorporated into the ninth edition, which has been in use for three years. German and Danish translations have been made.

3. COMPARABILITY OF THE VARIOUS EDITIONS

Since there has been a process of development and modification, the various editions of the PSE are not strictly comparable with each other, particularly not at the stage of item-ratings. However, items from the seventh and eighth editions are grouped into symptoms which are approximately comparable, although the item-composition of each symptom is not identical (see chapter 3). Once the symptoms are further grouped into syndromes (see chapter 4), even more comparability is assured and from that stage onwards, data from the seventh, eighth and ninth editions follow exactly the same path through the Catego procedure (see chapter 6).

The principles of interviewing have remained the same throughout the development of the PSE and those set out in the following section apply to the seventh, eighth and ninth editions. The principles of scoring do, however, differ somewhat between editions and those given below apply particularly to the ninth edition (as do the instructions concerning cut-off points). Special instruction is required in order to use the eighth edition.

4. PRINCIPLES OF INTERVIEWING AND SCORING

Basically, the schedule is a check list which systematically covers all the phenomena likely to be considered during a present state examination, and indicates how they are to be coded. Each of the items or symptoms is defined in greater or less detail. For most items or symptoms, a form of questioning is suggested, so that it would be possible to carry out the whole of the interview without deviating from the schedule at all. In practice, this would almost never happen since no two interviews are alike and the examiner must be able to adapt his technique to the situation. The wording of each question depends on the answer to the previous one. The principles for conducting the interview flexibly while preserving a substantial degree of stan-dardisation, which are described in this section, apply equally to all editions of the PSE. From a purely operational point of view, the term 'item' used in the eighth and earlier editions is correct but, for convenience, the term 'symptom' is used in the ninth.

I. THE INTERVIEW IS BASICALLY CLINICAL AND NOT A QUESTIONNAIRE

The schedule is laid out in question form to facilitate and standardise the interview, but each numbered question or item (together with suggested probes, in round brackets, and any other probes the examiner thinks necessary) represents a symp-tom; it is this symptom which should be rated as present or absent. A symptom should not be rated as present simply because the patient says 'yes'. A further description should be asked for, in the patient's own words, and further specific questions asked as necessary. Following this process of cross-examination (which can almost always be made acceptable to the patient), the examiner should make up his own mind as to how the symptom should be rated. Similarly, the fact that the patient says 'no' to the standard question does not mean that the symptom must be rated as absent. All available cues, in behaviour and case-record, and from all parts of the interview, should be used to determine whether a particular line of exami-nation should proceed further.

II. THE TIMING AND TIME SCALE OF THE INTERVIEW

The time period covered is one month before the interview. During the development stage, periods of three months and one week were tried out, as was a purely 'present state' interview. The last of these alternatives was least satisfactory since the time of most intense subjective experience of the symptoms was often a week or two before interview; that is, before the patient had contacted the service. Similarly, one week was often too short a period. On the other hand, many patients found it difficult to cover a period as long as three months without constant reminders. One month appeared to be a comfortable period to keep in mind. No doubt for special purposes a shorter or a longer period would need to be specified (if examinations were to be conducted at weekly intervals for example) but the schedule itself is written in terms of one month. Although this time scale is not specified in every question, it should always be understood and extra questions should be inserted from time to time in order to be sure that the patient is only describing the time period laid down. Some symptoms are labelled OE (on examination) and refer only to the condition observed by the examiner personally. Events which took place more than one month before the interview should be disregarded for purposes of rating the 'present state' but they are conveniently noted in the schedule for easy reference when the history is taken. In particular, it is not necessary to insist too rigidly on this criterion during the introductory section when the patient is giving an overview of his symptoms. A rough chronology should, however, be established.

It should be noted that the effect of limiting the period covered to four weeks is to exclude from consideration certain traits which can only be assessed on the basis of a much larger knowledge of the subject's attitudes, behaviour and reactions. Thus personality disorders and mental retardation, for example, could not be evaluated on the basis of only four weeks in the subject's life. The PSE schedule is not intended to cover such conditions. It is, however, applicable to the neurotic or psychotic disorders which arise in people who are also thought to have personality disorders or intellectual retardation.

The interview is intended to be carried out when an episode of symptoms is at its most intense (e.g. within a few days of admission to hospital), or at least when this peak of intensity falls within the previous month. It may, however, be useful to carry out the examination at other times, for example to measure change in symptomatology. A census investigation would, of course, discover many people not currently in an episode of symptoms.

It is perfectly acceptable for the interview to be carried out in two or even three stages if necessary, for example if the patient is too distressed or distractible or slow to complete it on one occasion. It is sometimes convenient to rate the behavioural sections in one session, e.g. when the patient is excited, and the subjective sections later.

A crude method for standardising the clinical history, in terms of the present and previous episodes and including possible aetiological factors, is described in chapter 4.

III. ORDER OF QUESTIONING

The introductory section is designed to give an overview of the 'present state' symptomatology and to provide a spontaneous sample of speech on which to judge disorders of form, stream and content. It also provides an opportunity to rate the patient's response to questions and relationship with the interviewer. It is not essential that the patient's account during this phase should stay strictly within the one month period. A rough chronology should, however, be established and the patient brought back to relatively recent events before starting the more structured part of the interview.

For psychotic patients, it will usually be convenient to proceed straight from the introductory section to sections dealing with hallucinations and delusions, returning later to the section on worrying.

Most patients with non-psychotic conditions can give a fair account with very little prompting and it is usually convenient to proceed straight to the section on worrying, thereafter following the section order suggested in the schedule.

However, the main principle is that the interviewer should be flexible. If it seems convenient, for example, to proceed from symptom 31 in the ninth edition (simple ideas of reference) to symptom 72 (delusions of reference), and then return to symptom 32, it is perfectly legitimate to do so. The order must be dictated by the overriding need to obtain full and accurate information.

If the interview is long or difficult, it is best to cover the most important sections first; it does not then matter so much if it is impossible to complete everything in one sitting. It may be perfectly legitimate to complete the schedule in two or even more sessions of interviewing, particularly if the main reason for using the PSE is to make a diagnosis.

IV. CUT-OFF POINTS

The cut-off point is another feature derived from ordinary clinical interviewing. Most sections contain a number of questions which are asked of everyone but if there is no indication whatever, from any source, that further questioning will be productive, a tick may be placed in the cut-off box and the questions below that point omitted. The section on delusions has only one cut-off point although there are many subsections, so it is particularly important to be quite sure that there is no likelihood of delusions being present, when cutting-off.

The examiner should *always* proceed beyond the cut-off point if there is any evidence (or any doubt) about a symptom below that point being present. If there is no such evidence, and no doubt in the examiner's mind that it would be a waste of time to ask the remaining questions, a tick should be placed in the cut-off box and the questions below the line omitted. Symptoms below the cut-off point will then automatically be scored as absent. The ninth edition has a 'secondary cut-off system' which is explained in the preamble to the schedule itself.

V. GENERAL PROBES

General probes, such as 'Could you tell me more about that?' are not specified in the schedule but the examiner may use them at any point, and should do so if he is in any doubt as to the nature of the phenomena. It has already been emphasised that each question represents a symptom and considerable cross-examination (which cannot be laid down in the schedule) may be necessary to establish whether the symptom is present or not.

VI. WORDING OF QUESTIONS

The criterion aimed at is a good clinical interview, with good rapport with the patient. The suggested form of words should be adhered to as far as possible, consistent with this criterion.

VII. NEGATIVE FORM OF QUESTIONS

Negative questions should be avoided whenever possible; for example, the form 'You don't hear voices?' should not be used. Occasionally it is necessary to phrase some questions this way because of the patient's hostile attitude to imputations that abnormalities might be present – a negative form might then bring out pathology where the usual questions would lead to termination of the interview. Negative forms may also be used to vary a form of questioning which appears to be getting monotonous, but only when the examiner is satisfied that the patient will not be unduly influenced. Apart from such occasions, the form of questioning should follow that laid down in the schedule.

VIII. EACH SYMPTOM SHOULD BE RATED ON THE WHOLE INTERVIEW

The examiner should always go back over the schedule and modify any ratings as necessary in the light of information elicited during the rest of the interview, after the original ratings were made. During training, the interview should be tape-recorded so that the ratings can be checked at leisure. Ratings should *always* be completed as the interview proceeds; subsequent reviews are for checking details, and alterations should not often be necessary.

IX. EXAMPLES OF SYMPTOMS

It is desirable to note on the schedule an example of any symptom which is rated as present. This is most important, since it is often quite difficult to remember, later on, why a particular symptom was rated. It is also most useful in analysis.

X. SCORING OF SYMPTOMS

Most symptoms are scored 0, 1, 2, 8 or 9. (0) means that the symptom was absent during the past month, (8) that the examiner is not sure even after proper enquiry whether the symptom has been present during the past month, and (9) that no decision can be made because the question was not asked or the patient did not answer or replied incomprehensibly. If the cut-off box is ticked, however, the symptoms below the cut-off point are automatically rated (0). Instructions concerning scoring (0), (1) or (2) are given in the preamble to the glossary of definitions of symptoms.

XI. SECTIONS

The questions are divided into sections for convenience only. The titles of sections have no diagnostic significance. Sections are not mutually exclusive and patients can be given ratings on symptoms from any combination of sections; for example, elation and depression may both have been present during the previous month.

XII. CASE-RECORDS AND OTHER INFORMATION

When the PSE is being used to arrive at the best information possible, it is sensible for the examiner to be well-prepared for the interview by reading any case-records available. Such material should only be used in framing questions, and will thus lead to a more general coverage. It should not, of course, be allowed to predetermine the ratings. For example, if the case-record states that a patient is certainly deluded, but there is no evidence of this in the interview and the patient denies any delusion during the past month, a rating of 9 (= not sure) should be made, or even (0), if the examiner thinks the case-note mistaken. In no case should a rating of (1) or (2) be made solely because of something recorded in case-notes. This will be taken into account in a different way (see chapter 4).

There are other circumstances, however, in which reading the case-notes might prejudice a study; for example, when the diagnosis of the clinician writing the case-notes is to be compared with the diagnosis based on the PSE.

3

DERIVATION OF 'SYMPTOMS' AND CONSTRUCTION OF THE NINTH EDITION

1. DERIVATION OF THE SYMPTOMS FROM THE SIXTH, SEVENTH AND EIGHTH EDITIONS

From the earliest versions of the PSE to the eighth edition there was a gradual increase in the number of items included. This was partly due to suggestions for further items as the schedule became increasingly widely used, but there had always been an intention in the early stages of development to have a large number of items rather than risk omitting something important. Analysis of the data from the large studies completed with the eighth edition indicated that the stage had been reached where little further needed to be added and that, in any case, condensation of the 500 or so items was necessary for a variety of statistical analyses. The need for some form of computer program that would give a completely reliable imitation of the clinical diagnostic process was the main motive behind this stage of the work, but other analyses such as clustering, further reliability studies, and factor analyses were also envisaged once the data had been condensed to a more manageable size.

Decisions about the original content and subsequent changes in the various editions of the PSE up to the eighth had always been clinical, and this principle was continued. The three main users of the eighth edition of the PSE, the IPSS, the MRC Social Psychiatry Unit and the US–UK Diagnostic Project, were all engaged at roughly the same time on a condensation of the items, so it was possible to take a great deal of experience into account in arriving at the 'symptoms' upon which Catego, the ninth edition, and various other analyses have subsequently been based. There are, no doubt many other ways in which the items could be clustered and used (Fleiss, Gurland and Cooper, 1971). The 'units of analysis' described in volume 1 of the International Pilot Study of Schizophrenia (WHO, 1973), although derived independently and by a different method, are very similar in item composition.

The main criteria for grouping the items together were similarity of content and infrequency. For instance, in the eighth edition there are nine items concerned with worrying which differ only in content; some patients worry about their health, others about their family, others about specific personal problems, others worry about all these things. All the items concerned with worrying were therefore grouped together and the ratings summed to give a score. A threshold score of 2 was then determined and anyone who reached this was assumed to have the symptom 'worrying'.

Another example may be given from the eighth edition. The symptom, 'delusions of control', is made up of eight items, each of which can be scored (0), (1) or (2). Thus the maximum score, if all items were rated (2), was 16. The threshold score was 2, so that if any one item was rated (2) or if any two were rated (1), the symptom was regarded as present. In this particular case, a rating of (1) on only one item might still carry considerable clinical significance and special instructions were included in the computer program to deal with the various contingencies that might arise (see chapter 6). In general, however, scores below threshold level were ignored and the symptom is regarded as absent. The frequency counts of items in the US–UK series were examined and items which were very rarely used were grouped with commoner ones of the same type. In this way, 145 'symptoms' were constructed and a computer program was written for each of the main editions using items as input and having a list of symptoms (list I) as the end-point.* All versions of the seventh and eighth editions therefore became comparable in terms of symptom list I.

The term 'symptom' is defined in the rest of this monograph in this purely operational way. The item composition of the symptoms in list I, and the frequency of occurrence of each one in the US–UK Diagnostic Project series (see chapter 7) is presented in appendix 3.1.

2. NINTH EDITION SYMPTOMS

It was decided that the symptoms derived in this way from the earlier editions of the schedule should be used as the basis for the ninth edition, and that they should be rated directly instead of through items. Most of the earlier item questions are retained but those that might be repetitive are placed in round brackets so that, once a symptom is established as present, it is not necessary to continue with that particular line of questioning. On the other hand, if there is any doubt, all the relevant questions must still be asked. Thus there is only one symptom of 'worrying' but many of the earlier item questions remain as probes or extra questions. The symptom 'delusions of control' is now rated as a unit but the earlier items are represented by questions in round brackets.

The opportunity was taken to make some revisions in list I, mainly by omitting a number of symptoms which were rarely used in the earlier analyses and appeared redundant. For example, the symptom 'auditory hallucinations from the body' (no. 95 in list I) was present very rarely and tended to be misunderstood by raters. It was therefore omitted. In other cases, a further condensation was made, for example, 'apprehension' and 'acute anxiety' (nos. 9 and 10 in list I) were combined to give the single symptom of 'subjective anxiety'. In a few cases, list I symptoms were divided into two units; for example, symptom 116 in list II ('nihilistic delusions') was split into two separate symptoms – 'hypochondriacal delusions' and 'delusions of catastrophe'. Finally, there was an important change in the rating of

---

* This formed stage 1 of the Catego program. See chapter 6.

auditory hallucinations based upon the observation in the analysis of IPSS and US–UK data that several different symptoms had been compressed into one. Affectively based and subculturally based hallucinations need to be separated from the rest.

In these ways, a new set of symptoms was derived which will be called list II. The differences between lists I and II are summarised in appendix 3.2.

The main difference between the ninth edition and the earlier ones is that the 140 list II symptoms are rated directly and the schedule can be completed rather more rapidly, to the extent that it is possible to decide on the presence or absence of symptoms without asking all the questions in brackets. In some cases the saving in time is very considerable, while in others there is very little difference between the eighth and ninth editions. In general, however, the eighth edition takes on average one hour, while the ninth edition takes about a quarter of an hour less. It is doubtful whether it is possible to make any further reduction (e.g. by decreasing the number of questions in brackets) without reducing the value of the schedule as a guide to a general 'present state' interview.

3. GLOSSARY OF DEFINITIONS

A major advantage of the ninth edition is that each symptom has been further described in a glossary, utilising experience with the earlier editions to emphasise points of differentiation which tend to be overlooked. Training with this glossary is essential if the ratings of symptoms are to be made in a uniform manner. In order to ensure uniformity when using this system, the definitions in the glossary are given as clearly as possible and they may therefore appear dogmatic. The aim, however, is simply to ensure ratings which are comparable even when made by psychiatrists from different schools of thought. It has been found that most clinicians can, with some training, use the criteria laid down even when they would not ordinarily do so in their own clinical practice. They do not thereby sacrifice the independence of their views in other clinical situations.

The ninth edition of the PSE and its glossary of definitions of symptoms will be found in a separate appendix at the end of the book. Separate copies are also available from Cambridge University Press.

4. SCREENING SCHEDULE DEVELOPED FROM THE NINTH EDITION

A version of the ninth edition, suitable for use in screening samples of the general population, has also been developed and is now under test. All the non-psychotic symptoms of the ninth edition are included, together with global ratings of certain psychotic symptoms. Studies currently being carried out will indicate whether this schedule, which has only fifty-four obligatory questions will be suitable for use in population screening by interviewers who are not medically qualified.

APPENDIX 3.1

DERIVATION OF SYMPTOMS FROM PSE ITEMS (EIGHTH EDITION)

Symptom number				Frequency of symptom in US–UK Series ($N = 688$)	Derivation from 8th edition	
List I (a)	(List II equiva- lent) (b)	Syndrome number (c)	Name of symptom (d)	(%) (e)	Item no. (f)	Item ratings (g)
1	(–)	(–)	Poor start	20.8	2.2 2.5	012 012 (4/1)*
2	(–)	(–)	Denial of worries	7.7	3.1	012 (2/1)
3	(4)	30 (WO)	General worry	58.9	3.2 3.3 3.4 3.5 3.6 3.8 3.9 3.10 3.11	012 012 012 012 012 012 012 012 012 (18/2)
4	(9)	34 (HY)	Hypochondriasis	11.9	3.7 3.12	012 012 (4/1)
5	(6)	30 (WO)	Tiredness	49.3	4A6	012 (2/1)
6	(7)	28 (TE)	Muscular tension	48.4	4A1 4A2 4A8	012 012 012 (6/2)

* (4/1) means that the maximum symptom score is 4 and the threshold is 1.

(a)	(b)	(c)	(d)	(e)	(f)	(g)
7	(5)	30 (WO)	Tension headache	29.8	4A7	012 (2/1)
8	(8)	28 (TE)	Restlessness	36.9	4A3 4A4 4A5	012 012 012 (6/2)
9	(11)	8 (GA)	Apprehension	28.8	4B1 4B4 4B6	012 012 012 (6/2)
10	(11)	8 (GA)	Acute anxiety	63.6	4B2 4B3	012 012 (4/1)
11	(-)	30 (WO)	Anxiety dreams	26.2	4B5	012 (2/1)
12	(14)	8 (GA)	Panic attacks	13.2	4B7	012 (2/1)
13	(15)	9 (SA)	Situational anxiety	14.4	4C1a 4C2a 4C3a 4C4a 4C5a 4C6a 4C7a	012 012 012 012 012 012 012 (14/2)
14	(17)	9 (SA)	Specific phobia	8.0	4C8a 4C8b	012 012 (4/1)
15	(18)	9 (SA)	Phobic avoidance	17.4	4C1b 4C2b 4C3b 4C4b 4C5b 4C6b 4C7b 4C9	012 012 012 012 012 012 012 012 (16/2)
16	(19)	6 (SD)	Inefficient thinking	46.0	5A1 5A2 5A3	012 012 012 (6/2)
17	(21)	30 (WO)	Neglect through brooding	17.3	5A4	012 (2/1)

(a)	(b)	(c)	(d)	(e)	(f)	(g)
18	(36)	29 (LE)	Subjective anergia	46.9	5B1 5B2 5B3 5B4	012 012 012 012 (8/2)
19	(28, 30)	32 (SU)	Social unease	46.6	5D1 5D2 5D3 5E2 5E3	012 012 012 012 012 (10/2)
20	(31)	27 (IR)	Ideas of reference	31.4	5C1 5C2	012 012 (4/1)
21	(32)	24 (ED)	Guilty ideas of reference	14.8	5C3	012 (2/1)
22	(29)	24 (ED)	Self-depreciation	25.4	5E1	012 (2/1)
23	(33)	24 (ED)	Guilt	–	5E5 12M1 12M2 12M3	012 012 01 01 (6/2)
24	(23)	6 (SD)	Depressed mood	68.2	5F1 5F2 5F3	012 012 012 (6/2)
25	(24)	6 (SD)	Hopelessness	57.1	5F4 5F5	012 012 (4/1)
26	(25)	6 (SD)	Suicidal plans or acts	15.0	5F6	012 (2/1)
27	(–)	6 (SD)	Gloomy thoughts	22.5	5F7 5F8	012 012 (4/1)
28	(–)	35 (OD)	Unvarying depression	16.7	5F9	01 (1/1)
29	(–)	35 (OD)	Special quality of depression	14.1	5F10	01 (1/1)
30	(26)	–	Depression or anxiety primary	15.7	4D12 5F14	012 012 (–)

(a)	(b)	(c)	(d)	(e)	(f)	(g)
31	(27)	35 (OD)	Morning depression	16.3	5F15	012 (1/1)
32	(–)	6 (SD)	Evening depression	16.4	5F16	012 (2/1)
33	(–)	35 (OD)	Poor appetite	37.5	5G1	012 (2/1)
34	(34)	35 (OD)	Loss of weight	44.5	5G2	012 (2/1)
35	(35)	30 (WO)	Poor sleep	55.9	5G4 5G5 5G6	012 012 012 (6/2)
36	(37)	35 (OD)	Early waking	20.3	5G7	012 (2/1)
37	(–)	35 (OD)	Constipation	22.4	5G8	012 (2/1)
38	(5)	35 (OD)	Depressive aches and pains	6.7	5G16	012 (2/1)
39	(38)	35 (OD)	Loss of libido	23.0	5G10	012 (2/1)
40	(–)	–	Increased libido	1.7	5G11	012 (2/1)
41	(39)	35 (OD)	Premenstrual tension	17.3	5G13	012 (2/1)
42	(40)	31 (IT)	Pent up anger	43.3	6.2 6.3	012 012 (4/1)
43	(40)	31 (IT)	Anger shown	51.9	6.1 6.4 6.5 6.6	012 012 012 012 (8/2)
44	(41)	12 (HM)	Subjective euphoria	11.3	7.2	012 (2/1)
45	(42)	12 (HM)	Subjective ideomotor pressure	12.9	7.1 7.3 7.5 7.11 9A3	012 012 012 012 012 (10/2)

(a)	(b)	(c)	(d)	(e)	(f)	(g)
46	(43)	12 (HM)	Grandiose ideas	7.3	7.4	012
					7.6	012
					7.7	012
					7.8	012
					7.9	012
					7.10	012
						(12/2)
47	(44)	7 (ON)	Checking and repeating	7.4	8.1	012
					8.5	012
					8.6	012
						(6/2)
48	(45)	7 (ON)	Obsessional cleanliness	6.0	8.2	012
					8.3	012
						(4/1)
49	(46)	7 (ON)	Other obsessions	9.7	8.7	012
					8.8	012
					8.9	012
					8.10	012
						(8/2)
50	(–)	–	Changed interests	1.7	9A4	012
						(2/1)
51	(22)	33 (IC)	Loss of interest	40.8	9A1	012
					9A2	012
					9A5	012
					9A6	012
					9A7	012
						(10/2)
52	(20)	33 (IC)	Poor concentration	48.7	9B1	012
					9B2	012
					9B3	012
					9B4	012
						(8/2)
53	(47)	23 (DE)	Derealisation	13.7	10.1	012
					10.4	012
						(4/1)
54	(54)	24 (ED)	Lost affect	15.4	10.3	012
						(2/1)
55	(48)	23 (DE)	Depersonalisation	11.6	10.2	012
					10.5	012
					10.6	012
					10.7	012
					10.9	012
					10.10	012
						(12/2)

(a)	(b)	(c)	(d)	(e)	(f)	(g)
56	(49)	22 (NP)	Unfamiliarity	5.8	11.2	012 (2/1)
57	(50)	22 (NP)	Heightened perception	3.9	11.3 11.5	012 012 (4/1)
58	(51)	24 (ED)	Dulled perception	2.8	11.4	012 (2/1)
59	(53)	–	Deja vu	3.2	11.8	012 (2/1)
60	(52, 53)	22 (NP)	Changed perception	5.2	11.1 11.6 11.7 11.11 11.12 11.13	012 012 012 012 012 012 (12/2)
61	(–)	–	Subjectively poor memory	31.8	9B5	012 (2/1)
62	(100)	10 (HT)	Brief amnesias	8.9	– (–)	
63	(103)	36 (OR)	Objectively poor memory	8.3	– (–)	
64	(104, 105)	–	Loss of insight	41.1	14.1 14.2 14.3 14.4	012 012 012 012 (10/2)
65	(95)	–	Preoccupation with delusions	36.5	12Q3	012345 (–)
66	(108)	26 (NG)	Self-neglect	14.5	15A1	012 (2/1)
67	(109)	–	Odd appearance	1.5	15A2	012 (2/1)
68	(110)	21 (SL)	Slow and underactive	12.9	15A3 15A4 15A5 15A8 15A10	012 012 012 012 012 (10/2)
69	(130)	21 (SL)	Slow speech	16.1	15A6 15A7	012 012 (4/1)

(a)	(b)	(c)	(d)	(e)	(f)	(g)
70	(94)	22 (NP)	Evasiveness	8.7	12Q2 17.8 18.6	012 012 <u>012</u> (6/2)
71	(111)	25 (AG)	Agitation	16.3	15B1 15B2 15B3 15B4	012 012 012 <u>012</u> (8/2)
72	(112)	20 (OV)	Gross excitement	1.6	15B5 15B6	012 <u>012</u> (4/1)
73	(113)	20 (OV)	Irreverent behaviour	3.2	15B7 16.17	012 <u>012</u> (4/1)
74	(131)	–	Too much speech	7.7	15B8 17D1 17D6	012 012 <u>012</u> (6/2)
75	(114)	–	Distractibility	5.2	15B9	<u>012</u> (2/1)
76	(115)	20 (OV)	Embarrassing behaviour	1.9	15C1 15C2	012 <u>012</u> (4/1)
77	(116)	2 (CS)	Mannerisms and posturing	2.9	15C7	<u>012</u> (2/1)
78	(117)	–	Other odd movements	3.8	15C8 15C9	012 <u>012</u> (4/1)
79	(118)	4 (RS)	Behaves as if hallucinated	1.3	15C10 15C12	012 <u>012</u> (4/1)
80	(119)	2 (CS)	Catatonic movements	2.3	15C13 15C14 15C15 15C16 15C17 15C18 15C20 15C21	012 012 012 012 012 012 012 <u>012</u> (16/1)

(a)	(b)	(c)	(d)	(e)	(f)	(g)
81	(120)	8 (GA)	Observed anxiety	16.4	15A9	012
					16.1	012
					16.2	012
					16.7	012
					16.32	012
						(10/2)
82	(121)	6 (SD)	Observed depression	14.2	16.3	012
					16.4	012
					16.8	012
					16.10	012
					16.11	012
					16.31	012
						(12/2)
83	(122)	–	Histrionic	2.5	16.14	012
						(2/1)
84	(123)	12 (HM)	Hypomanic affect	7.6	16.5	012
					16.15	012
					16.16	012
						(6/2)
85	(124)	31 (IT)	Hostile irritability	10.5	15C19	012
					16.18	012
					16.19	012
					16.20	012
					16.21	012
					18.7	012
						(12/2)
86	(125)	22 (NP)	Suspicious	6.0	16.22	012
						(2/1)
87	(126)	22 (NP)	Perplexed	10.8	16.23	012
						(2/1)
88	(49)	22 (NP)	Delusional mood	14.7	16.24	012
					12P10	01
						(3/1)
89	(127)	–	Labile mood	4.8	16.25	012
					16.26	012
						(4/1)
90	(128)	11 (AF)	Blunted affect	16.7	16.6	012
					16.9	012
					16.27	012
					16.28	012
						(8/2)
91	(129)	22 (NP)	Incongruity of affect	2.3	16.29	012
						(2/1)

(a)	(b)	(c)	(d)	(e)	(f)	(g)
92	(–)	–	Giggling to self	5.4	16.30	012
						(2/1)
93	(–)	13 (AH)	Auditory hallucinations	13.9	12A1	012
						(2/1)
94	(65)	13 (AH)	Pseudohallucinations	4.4	12A2	012
					12A3	012
						(4/1)
95	(–)	1 (NS)	Auditory hallucinations from body	2.8	12A6	012
						(2/1)
96	(63)	13 (AH)	Voices to patient	11.0	12A9 (omit 2)	01
						(1/1)
97	(62)	1 (NS)	Voices about patient	5.5	12A9 (omit 1)	0(2 = 1)
						(1/1)
98	(62)	1 (NS)	Commentary by voices	5.5	12A13	012
					12A14	012
					12A15	012
					12A16	012
						(8/2)
99	(55–58)	1 (NS)	Subjective thought disorder	10.9	12B1	012
					12B2	012
					12B3	012
					12B4	012
					12B5	012
					12B6	012
					12B7	012
					12B8	012
					12B9	012
						(18/2)
100	(59)	17 (SF)	Delusion of thought reading	3.8	12B18	012
					12B19	012
						(4/1)
101	(71)	1 (NS)	Delusions of control	7.1	12C1	012
					12C2	012
					12C3	012
					12C4	012
					12C5	012
					12C6	012
					12C7	012
					12C8	012
						(16/2)

(a)	(b)	(c)	(d)	(e)	(f)	(g)
102	(72)	15 (RE)	Delusions of reference	12.5	12F1	012
					12F3	012
					12F11	012
					12F12	012
					12F13	012
						(10/2)
103	(73)	15 (RE)	Delusions of misinterpretation	10.8	12F2	012
					12F4	012
					12F5	012
					12F6	012
					12F7	012
					12F10	012
					12F14	012
						(14/2)
104	(74)	14 (PE)	Persecution by people	19.9	12G1	012
					12G2	012
					12G3	012
					12G4	012
					12G7	012
					12G8	012
						(12/2)
105	(74)	14 (PE)	Other delusions of persecution	5.8	12F8	012
					12G6	012
					12G9	012
					12G10	012
						(8/2)
106	(75)	–	Delusions of assistance	2.8	12G13	012
						(2/1)
107	(76)	16 (GR)	Delusions of grandiose ability	5.4	12H1	012
					12H2	012
					12H4	012
					12H9	012
					12H11	012
						(10/2)
108	(77)	16 (GR)	Delusions of grandiose identity	2.3	12H3	012
					12H5	012
					12H6	012
					12H8	012
					12H10	012
						(10/2)

(a)	(b)	(c)	(d)	(e)	(f)	(g)
109	(78)	16 (GR)	Religious delusions	5.7	12J1	012
					12J2	012
					12J3	012
					12J4	012
					12J5	012
						(10/2)
110	(83)	17 (SF)	Culturally specific delusions	–	12J10	012
						(2/1)
111	(87)	17 (SF)	Fantastic delusions	2.3	12K1	012
					12K2	012
					12K3	012
					12K4	012
					12K5	012
					12K6	012
					12K7	012
					12K8	012
						(16/2)
112	(86)	17 (SF)	Sexual delusions	1.2	12L1	012
					12L2	012
					12L3	012
					12L4	012
					12L6	012
					12L8	012
					12L9	012
						(14/2)
113	(85)	17 (SF)	Delusions of pregnancy	0.3	12L5	012
						(2/1)
114	(84)	17 (SF)	Morbid jealousy	0.4	12L7	012
						(2/1)
115	(88)	5 (DD)	Delusions of guilt	5.7	12M2	0 (2 = 1)
					12M3	0 (2 = 1)
					12M4	012
					12M5	012
						(6/2)
116	(90–92)	5 (DD)	Nihilistic	2.9	12M6	012
					12M7	012
					12M8	012
					12M9	012
					12M10	012
					12M11	012
					12M12	012
					12M13	012
						(16/2)

(a)	(b)	(c)	(d)	(e)	(f)	(g)
117	(66)	18 (SH)	Visual hallucinations	5.8	12D1	012
					12D3	012
					12D9	012
					12D10	012
					12D11	012
						(10/1)
118	(67)	36 (OR)	Delirious visual hallucinations	0.9	12D12	012
						(2/1)
119	(–)	–	Hypnogogic visual hallucinations	1.7	12D13	012
						(2/1)
120	(–)	–	Visual illusions	0.9	12D16	012
						(2/1)
121	(70)	18 (SH)	Tactile hallucinations	3.5	12D4	012
						(2/1)
122	(70)	18 (SH)	Somatic hallucinations	3.8	12D5	012
						(2/1)
123	(68)	19 (OH)	Olfactory hallucinations	6.7	12D6	012
						(2/1)
124	(70)	18 (SH)	Gustatory hallucinations	0.7	12D8	012
						(2/1)
125	(69)	19 (OH)	Delusions that patient smells	–	12D7	012
						(2/1)
126	(70)	18 (SH)	Somatic delusions	2.8	12E1	012
					12E2	012
					12E3	012
					12E4	012
					12E5	012
					12E6	012
					12E7	012
					12E8	012
					12E9	012
						(18/2)
127	(82)	–	Autochthonous delusions	4.9	12F18	1 only
					12G15	1 only
					12J8	1 only
					12K11	1 only
					12L13	1 only
						(5/1)

(*a*)	(*b*)	(*c*)	(*d*)	(*e*)	(*f*)	(*g*)
128	(–)	–	No affective reaction to delusions	13.7	12A27	2 only
					12B20	2 only
					12C17	2 only
					12E12	2 only
					12F19	2 only
					12G16	2 only
					12J9	2 only
					12K12	2 only
					12L14	2 only
						(9/2)
129	(139)	–	Misleading answers	4.9	17.1	012
					17.2	012
					17.3	012
					17.4	012
						(8/2)
130	(132)	4 (RS)	Non-social speech	4.1	17A1	012
					17A2	012
					17A3	012
					17A4	012
					17A5	012
						(10/1)
131	(133)	21 (SL)	Muteness	3.8	17B1	012
						(2/1)
132	(134)	21 (SL)	Restriction of quantity of speech	9.0	17B2	012
					17B3	012
					17B4	012
					17B5	012
					17B6	012
						(10/1)
133	(135)	3 (IS)	Neologisms	1.9	17C1	012
						(2/1)
134	(136)	3 (IS)	Incoherence of speech	6.8	17C2	012
					17C3	012
					17C4	012
					17C6	012
					17C7	012
					17C8	012
					17C16	012
						(14/2)
135	(–)	3 (IS)	Irrelevant speech	4.1	17C5	012
						(2/1)

(a)	(b)	(c)	(d)	(e)	(f)	(g)
136	(138)	11 (SS)	Poverty of content of speech	2.6	17C11	012
					17C12	012
					17C13	012
					17C14	012
					17C15	012
						(10/2)
137	(137)	12 (HM)	Hypomanic content of speech	5.1	17D3	012
					17D4	012
					17D5	012
						(6/1)
138	(–)	–	Quantity of auditory hallucinations	15.8	12A8	012
					12A11	012
					12A12	012
					12A18	012
					12A19	012345
						(13/2)
139	(–)	17 (SF)	Delusional explanation – general	14.7	12A21	012
					12B12	012
					12C11	012
					12F18	2+ = 2
					12G15	2+ = 2
					12J8	2+ = 2
					12K11	2+ = 2
					12L13	2+ = 2
						(16/2)
140	(–)	–	Delusional explanation – people	0.9	12A22	012
					12B13	012
					12C12	012
						(6/2)
141	(79)	–	Delusional explanation – extra-sensory	0.9	12A24	012
					12B15	012
					12C14	012
						(6/2)
142	(80)	–	Delusional explanation – machines	0.7	12A25	012
					12B16	012
					12C15	012
					12F9	012
						(8/2)
143	(78)	–	Delusional explanation – ghosts	0.4	12A23	012
					12B14	012
					12C13	012
						(6/2)

(a)	(b)	(c)	(d)	(e)	(f)	(g)
144	(–)	–	Delusional explana- tion – illness	0.7	12A26 12B17 12C17	012 012 012 (6/2)
145	(–)	–	Nuclear symptoms	1.9	12P1–10	01 (10/1)

APPENDIX 3.2

RELATIONSHIP BETWEEN LIST I AND LIST II SYMPTOMS

	List II (9th edition) symptom no. and name (a)	Syndrome no. (b)	List I (6th–8th editions) symptom no. (c)
1	Physical health (subjective estimate)	–	–
2	Physical health	–	–
3	Psychosomatic symptoms	–	–
4	Worrying	30 (WO)	3
5	Tension pains	28 (TE)	7
6	Tiredness	30 (WO)	5
7	Muscular tension	28 (TE)	6
8	Restlessness	28 (TE)	8
9	Hypochondriasis	34 (HY)	4
10	Nervous tension	30 (WO)	–
11	Subjective anxiety	8 (GA)	9 and 10
12	Anxious foreboding	–	–
13	Anxiety due to delusions	–	–
14	Panic attacks	8 (GA)	12
15	Situational anxiety	9 (SA)	13
16	Anxiety on meeting people	32 (SU)	–
17	Specific phobias	9 (SA)	14
18	Anxiety avoidance	9 (SA)	15
19	Inefficient thinking	6 (SD)	16
20	Poor concentration	33 (IC)	52
21	Neglect through brooding	30 (WO)	17
22	Loss of interest	33 (IC)	51
23	Depressed mood	6 (SD)	24
24	Hopelessness	6 (SD)	25
25	Suicidal plans or acts	6 (SD)	26
26	Anxiety or depression primary	–	–
27	Morning depression	35 (OD)	31
28	Social withdrawal	32 (SU)	19
29	Self-depreciation	24 (ED)	22
30	Lack of self confidence	32 (SU)	19

	(a)	(b)	(c)
31	Ideas of reference	27 (IR)	20
32	Guilty ideas of reference	24 (ED)	21
33	Guilt	24 (ED)	23
34	Loss of weight	35 (OD)	34
35	Delayed sleep	30 (WO)	35
36	Subjective anergia	29 (LE)	18
37	Early waking	35 (OD)	36
38	Loss of libido	35 (OD)	39
39	Premenstrual exacerbation	35 (OD)	41
40	Irritability	31 (IT)	42 and 43
41	Expansive mood	12 (HM)	44
42	Ideomotor pressure	12 (HM)	45
43	Grandiose ideas and actions	12 (HM)	46
44	Obsessional checking and repeating	7 (ON)	47
45	Obsessional cleanliness and rituals	7 (ON)	48
46	Obsessional ideas and rumination	7 (ON)	49
47	Derealisation	23 (DE)	53
48	Depersonalisation	23 (DE)	55
49	Unfamiliarity and delusional mood	22 (NP)	56 and 88
50	Heightened perception	22 (NP)	57
51	Dulled perception	24 (ED)	58
52	Changed perception	22 (NP)	60
53	Changed perception of time	22 (NP)	59 and 60
54	Lost affect	24 (ED)	54
55	Thought intrusion	1 (NS) ⎫	
56	Thought broadcast	1 (NS) ⎪	99
57	Thought echo and commentary	1 (NS) ⎬	
58	Thought withdrawal	1 (NS) ⎭	
59	Thoughts read	17 (SF)	100
60	(1) Music, tapping	22 (NP)	–
	(2) Muttering, whispering	4 (RS)	–
61	(1) Voice calling name	22 (NP)	–
	(2) Depressive hallucinations	5 (DD)	–
	(3) Hallucinations based on elation	–	–
62	Voices about patient	1 (NS)	97 and 98
63	Voices to patient	13 (AH)	96
64	(1) Subcultural hallucinations	37 (SC)	–
	(2) Dissociative hallucinations	10 (HT)	–
65	Pseudohallucinations	–	94
66	(1) Minor visual hallucinations	22 (NP)	–
	(2) Visual hallucinations	18 (VH)	117
67	Delirious visual hallucinations	36 (OR)	118
68	Olfactory hallucinations	19 (OH)	123
69	Delusion that patient smells	19 (OH)	125

	(a)	(b)	(c)
70	(1) Other minor hallucinations (2) Delusional elaboration of hallucinations	22 (NP) 17 (SF)	121, 122, 124 and 126
71	Delusions of control	1 (NS)	101
72	Delusions of reference	15 (RE)	102
73	Delusional misinterpretation and misidentification	15 (RE)	103
74	Delusions of persecution	14 (PE)	104, 105 and 140
75	Delusions of assistance	17 (SF)	106
76	Delusions of grandiose abilities	16 (GR)	107
77	Delusions of grandiose identity	16 (GR)	108
78	Delusional explanation (religious)	16 (GR)	109 and 143
79	Delusional explanation (hypnotism, etc.)	17 (SF)	100 and 142
80	Delusional explanation (physical forces)	17 (SF)	142
81	Delusional explanation (alien penetration	1 (NS)	–
82	Primary delusions	1 (NS)	127
83	Subculturally influenced delusions	37 (SC)	110
84	Morbid jealousy	17 (SF)	114
85	Delusions of pregnancy	17 (SF)	113
86	Sexual delusions	17 (SF)	112
87	Fantastic delusions	17 (SF)	111
88	Delusions of guilt	5 (DD)	115
89	Delusions concerning appearance	17 (SF)	–
90	Delusions concerning lack of organs	17 (SF)	–
91	Hypochondriacal delusions	5 (DD)	116
92	Delusions of catastrophe	5 (DD)	116
93	Systematisation of delusions	–	–
94	Evasiveness concerning delusions	22 (NP)	70
95	Overall preoccupation with delusions	–	65
96	Acting out delusions	–	–
97	Fugues, blackouts, amnesias	–	–
98	Drugs taken in past month	–	–
99	Alcohol abuse in past month	–	–
100	Dissociative states	10 (HT)	62
101	Conversion symptoms	10 (HT)	–
102	Clouding of consciousness or stupor	22 (NP)	–
103	Organic impairment of memory	36 (OR)	63
104	Insight (psychosis)	–	64
105	Insight (neurosis)	–	64
106	Social impairment (neurosis)	–	–
107	Social impairment (psychosis)	–	–
108	Self-neglect	26 (NG)	66
109	Bizarre appearance	22 (NP)	67

	(a)	(b)	(c)
110	Slowness and underactivity	21 (SL)	68
111	Agitation	25 (AG)	71
112	Gross excitement	20 (OV)	72
113	Irreverent behaviour	20 (OV)	73
114	Distractibility	–	75
115	Embarrassing behaviour	20 (OV)	76
116	Mannerisms and posturing	2 (CS)	77
117	Stereotypies	4 (RS)	78
118	Behaves as if hallucinated	4 (RS)	79 and 92
119	Catatonic movements	2 (CS)	80
120	Observed anxiety	8 (GA)	81
121	Observed depression	6 (SD)	82
122	Histrionic	10 (HT)	83
123	Hypomanic affect	12 (HM)	84
124	Hostile irritability	31 (IT)	85
125	Suspicious	22 (NP)	86
126	Perplexed	22 (NP)	87
127	Labile mood	–	89
128	Blunted affect	11 (AF)	90
129	Incongruity of affect	22 (NP)	91
130	Slow speech	21 (SL)	69
131	Pressure of speech	–	74
132	Non-social speech	4 (RS)	130
133	Muteness	21 (SL)	131
134	Restricted quantity of speech	21 (SL)	132
135	Neologisms	3 (IS)	133
136	Incoherence of speech	3 (IS)	134
137	Flight of ideas	12 (HM)	137
138	Poverty of content	–	136
139	Misleading answers	38 (DI)	129
140	Adequacy of interview	38 (DI)	–

List I symptoms not used separately in list II: 1, 2, 11, 27, 28, 29, 30, 32, 33, 37, 40, 50, 61, 95, 119, 120, 128, 138, 139, 144, 145

4

DERIVATION OF SYNDROMES: THE SYNDROME CHECK LIST

1. INTRODUCTION

Although the symptoms described in chapter 3 give a fairly complete profile of the phenomena likely to be observed during the present state examination of a patient with one of the functional psychoses or neuroses, and although the symptom profile is more easily comprehended than the data in the item-ratings, there is still too much information for ready consideration. A further data-reduction stage is therefore necessary. One way of doing this is to group together all symptoms of a similar kind, for example, anxiety–tension–irritability, depression–elation, etc. (WHO, 1973). However, if the symptom groups are to be used for classification it is important that specific diagnostic items should be kept apart. The symptoms were therefore grouped together into syndromes, using clinical judgement as the main criterion. The same syndromes were derived from the two lists of symptoms. Appendix 4.1 shows how the syndromes were derived from the ninth edition symptoms (list II) and appendix 4.2 gives the equivalent information for list I symptoms, together with the frequencies in the US–UK series. A common pathway is reached at the syndrome stage* and all recent versions of the PSE (seventh, eighth, US–UK, WHO and ninth editions) then become closely comparable. Certain changes have been made in the composition and derivation of syndromes from list II symptoms, based upon experience in use, but these are relatively small and unlikely to much affect comparability.

Table 4.1 gives the numbers, symbols and names of the syndromes. The symbols are mnemonics. The names, although they have diagnostic implications, are not at this stage in any way equivalent to diagnoses.

2. CHOICE OF SYNDROMES

There were three main reasons for grouping symptoms as shown in appendix 4.1. The most important was that the process of diagnosis requires a gradual reduction in the information available until finally only one or a few categorisations are made. This reduction must however, be done logically, combining like with like according to the rules of the diagnostic system being simulated. Thus syndrome 1 (NS) is composed of symptoms regarded by Schneider (1959, 1971) as 'first-rank', in the

---

* This is stage 2 of the Catego program. See chapter 6.

Table 4.1. *Symbols (mnemonics) used to label syndromes*

1	(NS)	Nuclear syndrome	21	(SL)	Slowness
2	(CS)	Catatonic syndrome	22	(NP)	Non-specific psychosis
3	(IS)	Incoherent speech	23	(DE)	Depersonalisation
4	(RS)	Residual syndrome	24	(ED)	Special features of depression
5	(DD)	Depressive delusions and hallucinations	25	(AG)	Agitation
6	(SD)	Simple depression	26	(NG)	Self-neglect
7	(ON)	Obsessional syndrome	27	(IR)	Ideas of reference
8	(GA)	General anxiety	28	(TE)	Tension
9	(SA)	Situational anxiety	29	(LE)	Lack of energy
10	(HT)	Hysteria	30	(WO)	Worrying, etc.
11	(AF)	Affective flattening	31	(IT)	Irritability
12	(HM)	Hypomania	32	(SU)	Social unease
13	(AH)	Auditory hallucinations	33	(IC)	Loss of interest and concentration
14	(PE)	Delusions of persecution			
15	(RE)	Delusions of reference	34	(HY)	Hypochondriasis
16	(GR)	Grandiose and religious delusions	35	(OD)	Other symptoms of depression
17	(SF)	Sexual and fantastic delusions	36	(OR)	Organic impairment
			37	(SC)	'Subcultural' delusions of hallucinations
18	(VH)	Visual hallucinations			
19	(OH)	Olfactory hallucinations	38	(DI)	Doubtful interview
20	(OV)	Overactivity			

sense that they are likely to be diagnostic of schizophrenia in the absence of organic features. These symptoms are distinguished from those in syndrome 13 (AH) because here the hallucinations are voices talking to the patient rather than about him. If this symptom is well enough defined (so that affectively or sub-culturally based hallucinations can be excluded), it is probably as indicative of schizophrenia as any in syndrome 1 (NS), but it is kept separate until the demonstration is made that it can be specifically rated. It is very simple, in the Catego program (see chapter 6), to group syndromes such as 1 (NS) and 13 (AH) together. It is difficult to separate them once they have been combined.

Similarly, it was considered on clinical grounds that, at this stage, it would be wise to separate a syndrome of simple depression, 6 (SD), from one of depressive delusions, 5 (DD), and others such as 21 (SL), 24 (ED), 29 (LE) and 35 (OD). The constituent symptoms can be redistributed in the light of the results but they would then have to be tested on another material. The same is true of syndromes such as hypomania, 12 (HM), grandiose and religious delusions, 16 (GR), delusions of persecution, 14 (PE), and overactivity, 20 (OV). At the syndrome stage the symptoms have been grouped together because they appear to be clinical units, whose diagnostic significance changes according to context. Thus the three syndromes 12 (HM), 16 (GR) and 20 (OV), together give a clear diagnostic picture of mania, but the three syndromes 13 (AH), 14 (PE) and 16 (GR) are likely to be diagnosed as schizophrenia. The main purpose of the syndrome stage is to form units upon which diagnostic rules can operate, according to the actual pattern of syndromes shown by an individual patient, in order to lead to a categorisation. This means that certain syndromes are deliberately conceived as 'rag bags', e.g. 22 (NP).

A second reason for deriving syndromes is to make possible descriptive profiles which will be comprehensible visually. Such profiles could be derived in many different ways – for example, all delusions could be placed together, or all disorders of perception, as in chapter 7 of the IPSS report. Syndrome scores might also be useful for describing change over time.

The third reason for constructing syndromes is that a brief method is needed for extracting clinical information from case-notes or other sources of historical clinical data about the patient. Sufficient detail is not usually available to allow symptom ratings, but the diagnostically more important syndromes could be rated on a syndrome check list.

3. STATISTICAL RELATIONSHIP BETWEEN SYMPTOMS AND SYNDROMES

The basis for deriving syndromes was clinical. It is also of interest to investigate the possibility of deriving syndromes according to purely statistical rules. The initial matrix however, is 140 x 140, and this exercise has not yet been carried out. It was, however, decided to make an *ex post facto* check on the syndromes already derived in order to discover whether each symptom was appropriately related to its allocated syndrome. The ratio used was the index of association in a two-way table:

		Syndrome	
		Absent	Present
Symptom	Absent	00	01
	Present	10	11

$$\text{Index of association} = \frac{n_{11}}{n_{10} + n_{01} + n_{11}}$$

The index is therefore the ratio between the number of cases in which both syndrome and symptom are present together and the number of cases in which either one or both are present. Cases in which neither syndrome nor symptom is present (often a very substantial proportion) are ignored.

The index of association was calculated between each of the 97 symptoms in list I which were used in the SCL, and each of the 35 syndromes, and the whole exercise was done twice, once using IPSS data and once using the US–UK series for

Table 4.2. *Relationship between each symptom and syndrome to which it is allocated; IPSS and US-UK material*

$$\text{Index of association} = \frac{n_{11}}{n_{10}+n_{01}+n_{11}}$$

Rank of index out of 35	IPSS	US–UK (Netherne–Brooklyn)
Highest	85	82
Second highest	10	6
Third to sixth highest	2	5
Not in first six	–	4
Total	97	97

replication. Table 4.2 shows that, using this index, most symptoms do have a satisfactory degree of association with the syndromes to which they are allocated.

Of the 97 symptoms used to construct syndromes, 85 in the IPSS series and 82 in the Netherne–Brooklyn series, show the highest index of association with the syndrome to which they have been allocated, rather than to the other 34 syndromes. The exceptions are presented in tables 4.3 and 4.4. No particular pattern emerges and the ratios are rarely so different that a strong case can be made for transferring the symptom to a different syndrome.

The index of association may not have sufficient discriminating power to be ideal for this purpose and the whole exercise was therefore repeated, using a different index:

$$\frac{\text{the probability of having syndrome } j \text{ when symptom } i \text{ is present}}{\text{the probability of having syndrome } j}.$$

In general, this analysis also confirms the present structure of syndromes. The main problem concerns depressive symptoms, since syndromes 6 (SD) and 24 (ED) overlap considerably, as do syndromes 29 (LE) and 35 (OD). A somewhat more rational structure could probably be derived both clinically and statistically. Further analysis will be undertaken with this in mind. Meanwhile, the syndrome list presented in appendix 4.1 will be retained since it is, in large part, confirmed and the changes suggested by the statistical analysis would not affect the results presented in later chapters of this manual except perhaps to improve them slightly. It does seem possible, however, that the subclassification of the depressions by the Catego program might benefit from a restructuring of syndromes 6, 24, 29 and 35.

Table 4.3. *Cases in which highest index of association (IA) is between a symptom and a syndrome to which it was not allocated clinically (IPSS series)*

Syndrome	Symptom	N	Syndrome with highest IA	IA	N with syndrome and symptom	Syndrome to which symptom is allocated (appendix 4.1)	IA	N with syndrome and symptom
1 (NS) N=472	95	63	13	0.14	63	1	0.13	63
	97	172	13	0.39	172	1	0.36	172
	98	137	13	0.31	137	1	0.29	137
4 (RS) N=214	130	60	2	0.32	38	4	0.27	59
6 (SD) N=959	26	74	24	0.09	41	6	0.08	74
17 (SF) N=646	111	57	16	0.16	45	17	(0.09	57)*
18 (SH) N=378	124	69	19	0.19	31	18	0.18	69
22 (NP) N=657	56	164	23	0.37	133	22	0.25	164
	57	115	23	0.27	96	22	0.18	115
	60	168	23	0.39	141	22	0.26	168
24 (ED) N=412	58	57	23	0.15	51	24	0.14	57
31 (IT) N=835	85	125	25	0.20	57	31	(0.15	125)*

* These ratios were fifth and sixth highest respectively. The rest were second highest.

Table 4.4. *Cases in which highest index of association is between a symptom and a syndrome to which it was not allocated clinically (Netherne–Brooklyn series)*

Syndrome	Symptom	N	Syndrome with highest IA	IA	N with syndrome and symptom	Syndrome to which symptom is allocated (appendix 4.1)	IA	N with syndrome and symptom
6 (SD)	26	54	24	0.16	35			*
	27	124	24	0.33	81	6	(0.31	124)†
8 (GA)	12	67	9	0.27	41	8	(0.20	67)†
	81	70	9	0.20	33	8	0.20	70
11 (AF)	136	11	3	0.17	5	11	(0.16	11)†
12 (HM)	46	25	16	0.43	13	12	0.23	25
	137	14	16	0.14	4	12	0.13	14
16 (GR)	108	1	20	0.13	1	16	0.06	1
21 (SL)	131	15	2	0.19	5	21	0.12	15
22 (NP)	57	18	17	0.17	5	22	(0.13	18)†
24 (ED)	21	61	27	0.30	49	24	0.30	61
	58	9	2	0.08	2			*
30 (WO)	7	139	32	0.34	95	30	(0.32	139)†
	17	48	29	0.17	43			*
31 (IT)	85	23	26	0.13	8			*

* Not in first six.   † Third, third, third, fourth and third respectively. The rest were second highest.

4. SYNDROME PROFILES

Each syndrome has a score, comprising the summed scores of its constituent symptoms, and a degree of certainty (0, ?, +, + +; see appendix 4.1). Syndrome profiles may be given, in terms of scores or degrees of certainty, for individual patients, or for groups of patients with some characteristic (such as diagnosis) in common.

In the latter case, mean standard scores may be used (with a fixed mean and standard deviation), or mean raw scores, or the proportion of patients in the group for whom the syndrome is present with a given degree of certainty (say + or ++). It should be noted that list I symptoms are defined in terms of a threshold score and that scores below the threshold point do not count towards syndrome scores.

Examples of syndrome profiles are given in chapter 7.

5. SYNDROME CHECK LIST

The list of syndromes given in appendix 4.1 can be used as a guide to rating episodes of illness in a manner comparable to that of the PSE. This means that the syndrome ratings can be compared with those derived from the PSE, can be fed into the later stages of the Catego program in order to reach a classification and can be combined together in various ways so as to give a complete picture of the dynamics of an illness over time. The rules of rating the syndrome check list are straightforward but conservative. Often the only data recorded are expressed very vaguely; 'patient is deluded and anxious', etc. Nothing can be made of such reports. However, when the clinical case-records are reasonably full or when an informant is at hand to give an account of past clinical history, excellent information may be available which it would be a pity not to include. It should, however, always be remembered that the degree of standardisation, and therefore of comparability, of data-collection is quite different to that attained from using the PSE. Due allowance can be made for this in interpreting the results.

The advantage of the syndrome check list (SCL), if good information is available, is that all the symptom definitions are already known to the clinician experienced in the PSE technique so that no further instruction is required except in the exercise of judgement concerning what to rate as present. The overriding rule is always to rate conservatively, never to give the benefit of the doubt and to rate according to specifics, not generalities. It is only worth rating the good information.

The main problem, apart from judgements about quality of data, is to separate the clinical history into episodes. Perhaps the most secure use of the SCL is to supplement a Present State Examination. In this case, the SCL is used to rate syndromes occurring during the present episode of illness, making use of all good-quality sources of information. The PSE allows the rating only of what the patient says about his symptoms during the previous month. For various reasons, this may not give a full coverage of the symptomatology. PSE and SCL together complete the clinical picture.

No rules are laid down for separating clinical episodes. The SCL may be used to cover one episode at a time or all similar episodes combined. This means that results should never be given unless the procedure used is fully described, otherwise a lack of comparability will be the result.

A small exercise was carried out during the IPSS project to assess the value of rating syndromes from the narrative case histories supplied by the nine Centres taking part, as a supplement to the PSE. The results are reported in chapter 7 and indicate that a degree of reliability and usefulness can be achieved even when the material available is limited and completely unstandardised.

APPENDIX 4.1

SYNDROMES DERIVED FROM SYMPTOMS IN NINTH EDITION OF PSE (LIST II) APRIL 1973 (SYNDROME CHECK LIST)

© Medical Research Council 1974
MRC Social Psychiatry Unit
Institute of Psychiatry
London SE5 8AF.

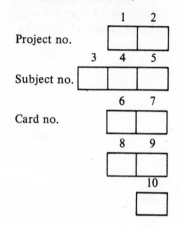

Project no.

Subject no.

Card no.

The syndromes formed out of the 140 symptoms rated in the ninth edition of the PSE are specified below, together with their symptom – composition. The presence of each syndrome may be directly rated from case-notes, interviews or other material concerning the clinical history, as well as derived from PSE ratings. Syndromes may be rated on the basis of the whole clinical history, each separate episode of illness, or the present episode. The period involved should always be specified. For the purposes of the Catego computer program, it is only necessary to rate syndromes 1–25. The others may, of course, be needed for other purposes.

When rating from case-records, always rate conservatively. Do not rate a syndrome present unless there is good evidence to this effect. For example, 'patient feels influenced' would *not* be sufficient evidence for 1 (NS). Write down an example whenever a positive rating is made. Use 8 (not known) freely. (9 = not applicable.)

Syndrome no. (a)	Syndrome name (b)	Symptoms (list II) (c)

| 1 (NS) | *Nuclear syndrome* | 55 Thought intrusion   62 Voices about patient
56 Thought broadcast   71 Delusions of control
57 Thought commentary   81 Delusions of alien penetration
58 Thought withdrawal   82 Primary delusions |

| | | 0 No symptoms
1 NS? = Partial delusions only   11
2 NS+ = 1 symptom
3 NS++ = 2+ symptoms |

| 2 (CS) | *Catatonic syndrome* | 116 Mannerisms and posturing
119 Catatonic movements |

| | | 0 No symptoms   12
2 CS+ = 1 symptom
3 CS++ = 2 symptoms |

| 3 (IS) | *Incoherent speech* | 135 Neologisms
136 Incoherence of speech |

| | | 0 No symptoms   13
2 IS+ = 1 symptom
3 IS++ = 2 symptoms |

| 4 (RS) | *Residual syndrome* | 60 (2) Hears muttering, whispering
118 Behaves as if hallucinated
132 Non-social speech |

| | | 0 No symptoms   14
2 RS+ = 1 symptom
3 RS++ = 2+ symptoms |

| 5 (DD) | *Depressive delusions and hallucinations* | 61 (2) Depressive hallucinations
88 Delusions of guilt
91 Hypochondriacal delusions (bowels blocked up)
92 Delusions of catastrophe |

| | | 0 No symptoms   15
2 DD+ = 1 symptom
3 DD++ = 2+ symptoms |

(*a*)	(*b*)	(*c*)

6 (SD)   *Simple*   19   Inefficient thinking
             depression   23   Depressed mood
                           24   Hopelessness
                           25   Suicidal plans or acts
                       121   Depression on examination

                                   0   No symptoms
                                   1   SD? = If no symptom 23 or 121
                                   2   SD+ = 1 symptom (23 or 121)
                                   3   SD++ = 2+ symptoms   **16**
                                           (including 23 or 121)

7 (ON)   *Obsessional*   44   Checking and repeating
              neurosis   45   Cleanliness and rituals
                           46   Obsessional ideas and rumination

                                   0   No symptoms   **17**
                                   2   ON+ = 1 symptom
                                   3   ON++ = 2+ symptoms

8 (GA)   *General*   11   Anxiety
              anxiety   14   Panic attacks
                        120   Anxiety on examination

                                   0   No symptoms   **18**
                                   2   GA+ = 1 symptom
                                   3   GA++ = 2+ symptoms

9 (SA)   *Situational*   15   Situational anxiety
              anxiety   17   Specific phobias
                           18   Anxiety avoidance

                                   0   No symptoms   **19**
                                   2   SA+ = 1 symptom
                                   3   SA++ = 2+ symptoms

10 (HT)   *Hysteria*   64   (2) Dissociative hallucinations (not
                                           subcultural)
                        100   Dissociative states
                        101   Conversion symptoms
                        122   Histrionic

                                 0   No symptoms   **20**
                                   2   HT+ = 1 symptom
                                   3   HT++ = 2+ symptoms

11 (AF)   *Affective*   128   Blunted affect   **21**
              flattening
                                 0   No symptoms
                                 2   AF+ = 1 symptom

(a)	(b)	(c)

| 12 (HM) | *Hypomania* | 41 Subjective euphoria
42 Ideomotor pressure
43 Grandiose ideas and actions
123 Hypomanic affect
137 Hypomanic content of speech |

0   No symptoms
1   HM? = If only symptoms 42, 43
        or 139
2   HM+ = 1 symptom (41 or 123)
3   HM++ = 2+ symptoms   22
        (including 41 or 123)

| 13 (AH) | *Auditory hallucinations* | 63 Voices to patient (not depressive)   23 |

0   No symptoms
2   AH+ = 1 symptom

| 14 (PE) | *Delusions of persecution* | 74 Delusions of persecution |

0   No symptoms
1   PE? = Partial delusions only   24
2   PE+ = 1 symptom

| 15 (RE) | *Delusions of reference* | 72   Delusions of reference
73   Delusions of mis-interpretation |

0   No symptoms
1   RE? = Partial delusions only
2   RE+ = 1 symptom   25
3   RE++ = 2 symptoms

| 16 (GR) | *Grandiose and religious delusions* | 76 Delusions of grandiose ability
77 Delusions of grandiose identity
78 Religious delusions |

0   No symptoms
1   GR? = Partial delusions only
2   GR+ = 1 symptom   26
3   GR++ = 2+ symptoms

(a)	(b)	(c)
17 (SF)	*Sexual and fantastic delusions*	59 Thoughts read 70 (2) Delusional elaboration of \ hallucinations 75 Delusions of assistance 79 Delusional explanation (hypnotism, etc.) 80 Delusional explanation (rays, etc.) 84 Morbid jealousy 85 Delusions of pregnancy 86 Sexual delusions 87 Fantastic delusions 89 Delusions concerning appearance 90 Delusions concerning lack of organs

0   No symptoms
1   SF? = Partial delusions only
2   SF+ = 1 symptom   27
3   SF++ = 2+ symptoms

| 18 (VH) | *Visual hallucinations* | 66 (2) Visual hallucinations   28 |

0   No symptoms
2   VH+ = 1 symptom

| 19 (OH) | *Olfactory hallucinations* | 68 Olfactory hallucinations
69 Delusion that patient smells |

0   No symptoms   29
2   OH+ = 1 symptom
3   OH++ = 2 symptoms

| 20 (OV) | *Overactivity* | 112 Gross excitement
113 Irreverent behaviour
115 Embarrassing behaviour |

0   No symptoms   30
2   OV+ = 1 symptom
3   OV++ = 2+ symptoms

| 21 (SL) | *Slowness* | 110 Slowness and underactivity
130 Slow speech
133 Muteness
134 Restriction of quantity of speech |

0   No symptoms
2   SL+ = Any other symptoms
       but muteness   31
3   SL++ = Muteness (133)

(a)	(b)	(c)
22 (NP)	*Non-specific psychosis*	49 Unfamiliarity and delusional mood 50 Heightened perception 52 Changed perception 53 Changed perception of time 60 (1) Hears music, tapping, etc. 61 (1) Hears voice calling name 66 (1) Minor visual hallucinations 70 (1) Other minor hallucinations 94 Evasiveness concerning delusions 102 Clouding or stupor 109 Bizarre appearance 117 Stereotypies 125 Suspicion 126 Perplexity 129 Incongruous affect

    0   No symptoms
    1   NP? = 1 symptom   32
    2   NP+ = 2 symptoms
    3   NP++ = 3+ symptoms

| 23 (DE) | *Depersonalisation* | 47 Derealisation
48 Depersonalisation |

    0   No symptoms   33
    2   DE+ = 1 symptom
    3   DE++ = 2 symptoms

| 24 (ED) | *Special features of depression* | 29 Self-depreciation
32 Guilty ideas of reference
33 Guilt
51 Dulled perception
54 Lost affect |

    0   No symptoms   34
    2   ED+ = 1 symptom
    3   ED++ = 2+ symptoms

| 25 (AG) | *Agitation* | 111 Agitation on examination |

    0   No symptoms   35
    2   AG+ = 1 symptom

| 26 (NG) | *Self-neglect* | 108 Self-neglect |

    0   No symptoms   36
    2   NG+ = 1 symptom

| 27 (IR) | *Ideas of reference* | 31 Ideas of reference |

    0   No symptoms   37
    2   IR+ = 1 symptom

(a)	(b)	(c)

28 (TE)   *Tension*   5 Tension pains
7 Muscular tension
8 Restlessness

    0 No symptoms   38
    2 TE+ = 1 symptom
    3 TE++ = 2+ symptoms

29 (LE)   *Lack of energy*   36 Subjective anergia   39

    0 No symptoms
    2 LE+ = 1 symptom

30 (WO)   *Worrying, etc.*   4 Worrying
6 Tiredness
10 Nervous tension
21 Neglect through brooding
35 Delayed sleep

    0 No symptoms   40
    2 WO+ = 1 symptom
    3 WO++ = 2+ symptoms

31 (IT)   *Irritability*   40 Irritability
124 Hostile irritability

    0 No symptoms   41
    2 IT+ = Symptom 40
    3 IT++ = Symptom 124

32 (SU)   *Social unease*   16 Anxiety on meeting people
28 Social withdrawal
30 Lack of self confidence

    0 No symptoms   42
    2 SU+ = 1 symptom
    3 SU++ = 2+ symptoms

33 (IC)   *Loss of interest and concentration*   20 Poor concentration
22 Loss of interest

    0 No symptoms   43
    2 IC+ = 1 symptom
    3 IC++ = 2 symptoms

34 (HY)   *Hypochondriasis*   9 Hypochondriasis   44

    0 No symptoms
    2 HY+ = 1 symptom

(a)	(b)	(c)

35 (OD)	*Other symptoms of depression*	27 Morning depression
		34 Loss of appetite
		37 Early waking
		38 Loss of libido
		39 Premenstrual exacerbation
		
		    0 No symptoms
		    2 SO+ = 1 symptom
		    3 SO++ = 2+ symptoms
			45

36 (OR)	*Organic impairment*	67 Delirious visual hallucinations
		103 Organic impairment of memory
		
		    0 No symptoms
		    2 OR+ = 1+ symptom
			46

37 (SC)	*'Subcultural' delusions or hallucinations*	64 (1) 'Subcultural' hallucinations
		83 'Subcultural' delusions
		
		    0 No symptoms
		    2 SC+ = 1+ symptom
			47

38 (DI)	*Doubtful interview*	139 Misleading answers
		140 Interview doubtfully adequate
		
		    0 No item
		    2 DI+ = 1 item
			48

Symptoms not used in SCL: 1, 2, 3, 12, 13, 26, 61 (3), 65, 93, 95–99, 104–107, 114, 127, 131, 138

APPENDIX 4.2

SYNDROMES DERIVED FROM LIST I SYMPTOMS (EIGHTH EDITION) AND THEIR FREQUENCIES

Syndromes (a)	Constituent symptoms (b)	Rules of formation (c)	Percentage frequency in US–UK series (N = 688) (d)
1 (NS)	95, 97, 98, 99, 101, 127	NS? = Partial del. only NS+ = 1 symptom NS++ = 2+ symptoms	18.2
2 (CS)	77, 80	CS+ = 1 CS++ = 2	4.5
3 (IS)	133, 134, 135	IS? = 1 IS+ = 2 IS++ = 3	8.9
4 (RS)	79, 130	RS+ = 1 RS++ = 2	5.1
5 (DD)	115, 116	DD+ = 1 DD++ = 2	7.1
6 (SD)	16, 24, 25, 26, 27, 32, 82	SD? = 1 SD+ = 2 SD++ = 3+	82.0
7 (ON)	47, 48, 49	ON? = 1 ON+ = 2 ON++ = 3	16.6
8 (GA)	9, 10, 12, 81	GA? = 1 GA+ = 2 GA++ = 3+	70.5
9 (SA)	13, 14, 15	SA? = 1 SA+ = 2 SA++ = 3	21.4
10 (HT)	62	HT+ = 1	8.9
11 (AF)	90, 136	AF+ = 1+	18.0
12 (HM)	44, 45, 46, 84, 137	HM+ = 1 HM++ = 2+	21.9

(a)	(b)	(c)	(d)
13 (AH)	93, 94, 96	AH+ = 1+	18.9
14 (PE)	104, 105	PE? = partial PE+ = 1 PE++ = 2	20.5
15 (RE)	102, 103	RE? = partial RE + = 1 RE++ = 2	15.6
16 (GR)	107, 108, 109	GR? = partial GR+ = 1 GR++ = 2	8.5
17 (SF)	100, 110, 111, 112, 113, 114, 139	AF? = partial SF+ = 1 SF++ = 2+	17.4
18 (SH)	117, 121, 122, 124, 126	SH? = 1 SH+ = 2 SH++ = 3+	10.8
19 (OH)	123, 125	OH+ = 1 OH++ = 2	6.7
20 (OV)	72, 73, 76	OV+ = 1 OV++ = 2+	5.7
21 (SL)	68, 69, 131, 132	SL+ = 68, 69 or 132 SL++ = 131	24.3
22 (NP)	56, 57, 60, 70, 86, 87, 88, 91	NP? = 1 NP+ = 2 NP++ = 3+	33.7
23 (DE)	53, 55	DE+ = 1 DE++ = 2	18.5
24 (ED)	21, 22, 23, 54, 58	ED+ = 1 ED++ = 2+	39.5
25 (AG)	71	AG+ = 1	16.3
26 (NG)	66	NG+ = 1	14.5
27 (IR)	20	IR+ = 1	31.4
28 (TE)	6, 8	TE? = 1 TE+ = 2	57.4
29 (LE)	18	LE+ = 1	46.9
30 (WO)	3, 5, 7, 11, 17, 35	WO? = 1 WO+ = 2 WO++ = 3+	84.2
31 (IT)	42, 43, 85	IT+ = 42 or 43 IT++ = 85	69.9
32 (SU)	19	SU+ = 1	46.5

(a)	(b)	(c)	(d)
33 (IC)	51, 52 .	IC+ = 1	
		IC++ = 2	58.4
34 (HY)	4	HY+ = 1	11.9
35 (OD)	28, 29, 31, 33, 34, 36,	OD? = 1	
	37, 38, 39, 41	OD+ = 2	
		OD++ = 3+	74.3
36 (OR)	63	OR+ = 1	8.7

5

THE RELIABILITY OF THE PSE AND
ITS RELATED DIAGNOSTIC PROCEDURES

1. INTRODUCTION

The development in the last few years of the PSE and of other standardising interviewing and rating procedures, such as the MSS (Spitzer *et al.*, 1964), the PSS
(Spitzer *et al.*, 1970), the IMPS (Lorr *et al.*, 1963) and the SPICS (Goldberg *et al.*,
1970) has radically changed the previously gloomy picture of the reliability of
psychiatric diagnosis noted in the 1960s by reviewers such as Kreitman (1961),
Zubin (1967) and Beck *et al.* (1962), at least from the viewpoint of research procedures. Recent experience with these standardised 'instruments' has shown that
the reliability of both description of symptoms and of the final choice of diagnosis
can rise to quite respectable levels. This chapter summarises the evidence on the
various aspects of reliability of the PSE and the related diagnostic procedures. Since
most of this evidence has been published elsewhere in detail, only the main points
will be dealt with. Some problems associated with the learning process are also
discussed.

The PSE is intended as an aid to reliable diagnosis, so it is necessary to consider
the reliability of the several stages of the diagnostic process that have been investigated when using it. The reliability of the following stages will be discussed: the
basic interview and ratings of items, section scores, Catego symptoms and syndromes,
IPSS 'units of analysis', diagnosis according to the categories developed with the
fifth, sixth and seventh editions of the PSE, and diagnosis according to the ICD-8.

Repeatability (defined as the reliability over short periods of time), the reliability
of observed behaviour, the learning process and consistent differences between
raters, or bias, will also be considered.

2. THE RELIABILITY OF THE BASIC INTERVIEW AND
RATINGS OF ITEMS

The PSE should be viewed as a first and fundamental step in a chain of stages, all of
which are needed to ensure that the diagnostician will be able to arrive at a reliable
diagnosis under clinical conditions. The first two steps are in fact contained within
the PSE schedule, and it is easy to forget that the PSE is composed of two closely
related but potentially separate procedures. First, there is the interviewing technique
composed of the style and the content of the questions, which allow the inter-

viewer to elicit the symptoms and draw his attention to any abnormal behaviour. In theory, the user of the PSE could learn this content and this way of questioning without making any attempt to rate the symptoms and behaviour so elicited. The second component consists of the descriptions and rules which indicate how the information elicited by the interview is to be recorded. It would be possible for an observer present at an interview or listening to a recording of an interview by someone else to learn to rate the items reliably without himself being able to conduct the clinical interview. In practice, both these components are regarded as complementary, and the interviewer learns to do both procedures at the same time.

The reliability of the interviewing technique itself, separated from the rating procedures, has not yet been studied, largely because it is most convenient to teach and learn both these components of the PSE together. Such a study would be difficult to undertake, because of the many subjective judgements that would be needed about personal styles of interviewing, and the appropriateness and number of optional extra probing questions. Judgements of this sort are, of course, made during the teaching of the interview, but are informal and are usually communicated as simple personal judgements such as 'too long-winded', 'too abrupt', 'not enough probes', 'sticking too close to the schedule', until the learner achieves a compromise between his own style, the restrictions of the schedule, the standards of the teachers, and the tolerance of patients.

The inter-observer reliability of ratings of individual items has been studied extensively by the US–UK Diagnostic Project and the World Health Organisation IPSS* and, with only minor exceptions, high levels of reliability have been achieved. Kendell *et al.* (1968) used the statistic *Kappa* (Cohen, 1968), to identify the least reliable items, and to compare the results of a reliability study with one on repeatability. The mean value of *Kappa* for all items was 0.77 in the reliability study (1.0 signifying perfect agreement and 0 only chance agreement), which was regarded as a satisfactory overall level, although the lack of similar studies in the literature for comparison make proper evaluation difficult. (*Kappa* has two advantages over more conventional measures; first, it is not affected by chance agreement, which varies with incidence, and second, a variation 'weighted *Kappa*' can be calculated which allows weights to be assigned to different degrees of disagreement so as to convey something of their relative importance.)

Item reliability was mainly studied in the IPSS by means of the 'intraclass correlation coefficient', a form of one-way analysis of variance (Hays, 1967). Tests of item reliability were carried out between nine Field Research Centres as well as simpler studies of inter-observer reliability on both live and video-taped interviews. The range of values of the intraclass correlation coefficient between centres was from 0.97 to 0.43, with a median of 0.77. These were regarded as acceptable values. Other methods were also used with similar results (Sartorius, Brooke and Lin, 1970; WHO, 1973).

* These two large-scale international projects are described further in chapter 7.

In all these detailed studies, some items were consistently more reliable than others, although, of course, items of very low reliability had been eliminated or improved during the progression through the earlier editions.

In general, items covering depressive symptoms have proved to be consistently very reliable, while items on anxiety are less so, with other types of symptoms variable and intermediate. The finer details and points of the comparative reliability also depend upon the design and size of the reliability study in question, and upon the method of analysis used.

3. THE RELIABILITY OF THE SECTION AND SYNDROME SCORES

The first report on the PSE (Wing *et al.*, 1967) was concerned principally with section scores, which are the sums of the scores for the items within each section; each section contains a fairly homogeneous group of items according to conventional clinical description. The composition of section scores changed very little during the progression from third to eighth edition, so that the results of this study can be considered together with those of Kendell *et al.* (1968) using the seventh edition and Wing (unpublished) using early IPSS data. Section scores have a very high inter-observer reliability in terms of the product-moment reliability coefficient; in both studies almost all the sections had a correlation coefficient between 0.80 and 0.95, with the situational anxiety section standing out as the lowest at 0.58. This high reliability might perhaps be expected, since two observers might arrive at the same section score, even though the ratings of the constituent items in that section were not the same. In spite of this, however, it is a very important level of reliability to study since the section scores, representing a summary of judgements over a homogeneous group of items, is probably a close approximation to the usual unstandardised judgements about severity of anxiety, depression, tension, etc. that are made in everyday clinical work.

The reliability of syndrome scores was tested on the IPSS material; 190 interviews were rated by two psychiatrists, one the interviewer and one an observer. Another fifty-one patients were interviewed twice. Product-moment correlation coefficients were calculated using the first thirty-five syndrome scores. The coefficients of reliability fell within the same range as those of the studies mentioned above but with a rather higher median value.

4. RELIABILITY OF 'UNITS OF ANALYSIS' AND GROUPED UNITS

The reliability studies reported in volume 1 of the IPSS were based upon 124 'units of analysis' which are very similar (and in many instances almost identical) to the Catego symptoms, although they were derived independently. The reliability of these units of analysis is high, and of the same order as the Catego syndromes and the original section scores. The IPSS results are of special interest because they allow the examination of reliability both within and between the nine Field Research Centres. The intraclass correlation coefficient for units of analysis within the centres had a range of 0.47 to 0.96, with a median of 0.81. Between centres, there was naturally a lower level, but still reaching acceptable levels in most instances (ranges 0.00–0.84, median 0.45).

Groups of units of analysis amalgamated on the basis of type of psychopathology (e.g. perceptual disturbances), were also studied. As for the other quantities, the reliability tends to rise as the information examined undergoes condensation. The within-centre intraclass correlation coefficient for the twenty-seven groups of units of analysis revealed many variations, some centres producing much higher values than others; the mean reliability for all the groups of units of analysis together for each centre ranged from 0.53 to 0.90, with a mean of 0.83. Again, the between-centre variation was greater, with a median value of 0.57, compared with a median of 0.84 for within-centre variation. These results, and the techniques of analysis used, are discussed in considerable detail in the IPSS report, and the overall conclusion was that they represent a satisfactory level of comparability, given the inevitable differences between the nine Field Centres.

5. THE RELIABILITY OF 'DIAGNOSIS' ACCORDING TO THE CATEGORIES DEVELOPED WITH THE FIFTH, SIXTH AND SEVENTH VERSIONS OF THE PSE

A list of simple descriptive categories tailored to the use of the PSE was developed as it went through the first five editions (Wing *et al.*, 1967). These categories are not complete diagnoses, since they utilise only information that might be expected to emerge from the PSE interview. These eleven categories, given below, are a rational means of testing the ability of the PSE by itself to aid in improving the reliability of the penultimate stage of the diagnostic process, before information about history and background is used. One hundred and seventy-two PSE interviews were categorised on this list by two psychiatrists (116 being inter-observer reliability comparisons and 56 being repeatability comparisons), and complete agreement was obtained in 84% of cases, partial agreement in 7% and disagreement in 9%. Table 5.1 shows the number of cases placed into eleven diagnostic groups by the first examiner, on the basis of PSE information only, and the number placed into exactly the same category by the second examiner.

Ten of the twenty-eight cases in which there was some measure of disagreement involved the notoriously difficult category of 'personality disorder' for which the PSE alone is not well suited.

Table 5.1. *Agreement on diagnostic category using PSE information only*

	First examiner	Second examiner	
'Schizophrenia (possible, probable or residual condition)'	75	69	(92%)
'Psychotic depression (possible or probable)'	15	12	(80%)
'Mania (possible or probable)'	4	4	
'Other functional psychoses'	2	2	
'Dementia (possible or probable)'	2	2	
'Non-psychotic depression (retarded)'	8	6	
'Non-psychotic depression (other)'	35	28	(80%)
'Anxiety state (general, situational or specific)'	17	13	(76%)
'Obsessional neurosis (possible or probable)'	2	2	
'Personality disorder'	6	3	
'No abnormality in present state'	6	3	
	172	144	(84%)

6. THE DIAGNOSIS ACCORDING TO THE INTERNATIONAL CLASSIFICATION OF DISEASES, EIGHTH REVISION

To make a full diagnosis according to an accepted standard classification, such as the ICD-8, needs more information than usually emerges from a mental state interview, so studies of this aspect of reliability involve much more than just the PSE. Personal, social and family history interviews with patients and relatives need to be taken into account, and the course of the illness itself may need consideration. Details of the IPSS and US–UK Diagnostic Project studies on these points may be found in the respective reports (Sartorius, Brooke and Lin, 1970; WHO, 1973; Cooper *et al.*, 1972), and show that, in general, high levels of reliability have usually been achieved.

7. REPEATABILITY

When a second interviewer carries out a repeat PSE interview within a day or so of the first, it is expected that there will be more and larger differences between the two sets of ratings than with an inter-observer reliability comparison, but even so the comparison of the two types of reliability is of importance. If very large differences in either symptom ratings or diagnoses were commonplace in such repeatability studies, the whole basis of the PSE and similar procedures would be called into question. In the event, only a moderate decrease in the various statistical values of reliability was recorded in all three repeatability studies that have been carried out. Kendell *et al*. (1968) found that, for items, *Kappa* decreased from a mean of 0.71 for inter-observer reliability to 0.41 for repeatability, whereas for section scores, *Kappa* fell from a mean of 0.84 to a mean of 0.64. In the IPSS studies and in the first study by Wing *et al*. (1967), similar changes were found. This degree of change seems reasonable, if it is remembered that not only is a different interviewer involved, with inevitable small differences in interviewing technique as well as in rating behaviour, but the patient is quite likely to show a real change in his symptoms and behaviour, as well as being likely to express himself differently on the two occasions.

8. THE RELIABILITY OF RATINGS OF OBSERVED BEHAVIOUR

Another consistent finding in all the PSE studies is the relatively low reliability and repeatability of judgements of observed behaviour, such as abnormal gait or movements, agitation and facial expression. This came as a surprise to most of the raters, since on *prima facie* grounds it might seem reasonable to suppose that such judgements could easily be dealt with by shared 'objective' criteria, as compared to the greater difficulty expected with the more 'subjective' reports by the patient of his own experiences. In practice, however, it quickly becomes apparent during the discussion of disagreements between ratings immediately after a joint interview that there are large and often surprising differences in the sensitivity levels or baselines for judgement of what is abnormal in behaviour. These baseline differences cannot easily be resolved by the usual discussion processes, and tend to persist. Perhaps the fact that the patient rarely complains about motor behaviour is important, since the rater is dependent upon his own ideas of what is abnormal. However, the major factor is probably the brief time-sample available during the time of the interview, since there is plenty of evidence to show that abnormal behaviour can be rated very reliably over longer time periods (Wing and Brown, 1970).

9. THE LEARNING PROCESS

Studies of the descriptions of the investigations carried out by the major users of the PSE should leave the reader in little doubt that a decision to use the PSE carries with it some important and often troublesome implications in terms of training procedures, and checks on reliability and repeatability. Without a planned programme of initial effort and subsequent checks, maximal standards of comparability will neither be reached nor maintained.

All the main PSE studies have used the same basic training procedures, consisting largely of repeated joint interviews, in which learner and teacher take turns to conduct the interview with successive patients. Each interview is followed immediately by a detailed discussion of interviewing technique and of the disagreements in ratings between the teacher and the learner. If done thoroughly, such a discussion takes almost as long as the interview itself, so most training sessions should occupy some two hours. Somewhere between ten and twenty such sessions spread over several weeks is usually found to be the minimal training needed to bring a learner up to the standards of an experienced interviewer; quite a large proportion of this effort goes into familiarisation with the schedule contents and order of questions, until finally it becomes possible to keep closely to the schedule (which literally is known by heart) while still maintaining a natural and easy manner of questioning, sympathetic comments and additional minor probes. Audio-tape recordings and video-tape recordings of interviews are an invaluable aid to this process, since learners can then compare their ratings with agreed versions compiled by one or more experienced interviewers. Whatever aids are used, however, there is no substitute for the detailed discussion with a teacher immediately after the ratings have been completed.

The training procedure described above was arrived at on rational but arbitrary grounds, and in fact surprisingly little systematic knowledge is available about this complicated learning process. The end results of learning rating procedures have been studied from the point of view of inter-rater reliability, about which there is now an extensive literature. 'Response styles', or measures of consistent bias between raters, have also been studied a good deal (Grosz and Grossman, 1968). The learning process itself, however, has not been given much attention, and we do not know the most rapid or most efficient methods to use when teaching a new rating technique. With this ignorance in mind, one study of the learning process was carried out by the US–UK Diagnostic project using the PSE (Von Cranach and Cooper, 1972), and it is sufficiently relevant to this discussion to make a brief summary worthwhile here.

During the development of the PSE, and particularly during the reliability studies already mentioned, a strong subjective impression was formed by the psychiatrists concerned that inexperienced raters at first usually rated at a higher level of abnormality than those they were trying to imitate. This impression stimulated our interest in following the progress of rating behaviour through a period of learning, and when a number of enquiries were received from psychiatrists not associated with the US–UK Diagnostic Project, the IPSS or the MRC Social Psychiatry Unit, who were interested in learning the PSE, an intensive week of instruction was planned. Eight psychiatrists of varying age and experience were assembled at the Institute of Psychiatry for one week. During this time they were all occupied full-time on a programme of video-tapes and live interviews, during which four experienced interviewers taught them the PSE procedures. A less intense but longer learning period would have been preferable, but the concentrated week had to be accepted for practical reasons. Live interviews formed the basis of the training process. For these, the learners were split into groups of three or four, and they all rated a patient who was being interviewed by one of the learners. A teacher was also present and rated the interview. After the interview was finished, the teacher and learners went systematically through their ratings, discussing all disagreements and difficulties. Some video-tapes were also used in this way, and the total of ten learning sessions for each of the eight learners was available to study changes in rating behaviour compared with the teacher present at each interview.

Several measures of agreement and disagreement were constructed for this study, and followed throughout the learning week. The one of special interest for this paper was a measure of bias, in which bias was defined as the tendency of the learner to rate consistently more or less abnormality than the teacher. The following bias score was calculated for each learner for each taped or live interview:

$$\text{learner's bias score} = 100 + \frac{\left(\begin{array}{l}\text{no. of items where learner} \\ \text{rates higher than teacher}\end{array} - \begin{array}{l}\text{no of items where teacher} \\ \text{rates higher than learner}\end{array}\right) \times 100}{\text{no. of items rated positive by both teacher and learner}}.$$

Thus a consistent tendency of the learner to rate more positive items or at a higher level than the teacher will produce for that interview a bias score of more than 100; a bias score of 100 means that learner and teacher's disagreements cancel out in terms of bias: and a bias score of less than 100 means that the learner rates consistently fewer items or at a lower level than the teacher. Figure 5.1 shows the mean bias scores for the eight learners over the whole week. (Session 8 is omitted from the neurotic section analysis, since, due to a misunderstanding, some of the learners did not rate the neurotic sections, which were covered at the end of a long interview dealing largely with delusions.) There is no group bias at the beginning of the week, but a strong positive bias appears in sessions 4, 5 and 6 ($t_4 = 2.99, P < 0.025$: $t_5 = 2.05, P < 0.05$ and $t_6 = 2.16, P < 0.05$, d.f. = 7). This bias is not produced by very large deviations in a minority of the learners, but is a consistent finding with only one or two of the eight deviating from the common pattern. The bias disappears in sessions 7, 9 and 10: the bias scores being distributed around the teachers' baseline as in sessions 1, 2 and 3. Finally in session 11 a negative bias ($t = 2.58$, $P < 0.025$, d.f. = 7) appears again. Although on this last section the bias is small it is nevertheless significant, due to the small standard deviation.

One reasonable interpretation of these changes is that as the learners made a conscious effort to adopt the standards of the teachers, they became too sensitive; this was followed by a compensatory swing to a negative or insensitive bias, but with a diminished standard deviation as they became more experienced and consistent. We do not know to what extent these findings can be generalised, or how much they were dependent upon the individuals and the unusually concentrated programme. Over a longer period or a greater number of sessions, perhaps several oscillations about the agreed standard would have occurred.

Another point of importance is that in this group of comparatively senior

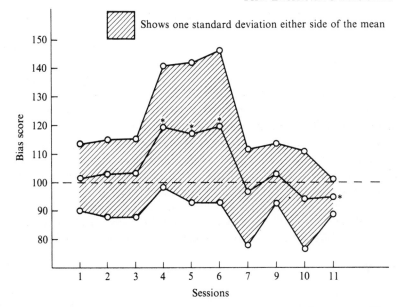

Figure 5.1. Mean bias score of eight learners over eleven sessions. Significance of difference between mean and 100 level is shown by * ($P < 0.05$).

psychiatrists, all achieved a satisfactory standard of agreement within the week allowed. But they were self-selected, and it could be that psychiatrists with less experience or different motives would not have learned so quickly. The ability to learn and use a set of criteria laid down by someone else may not be universal, and it may be that as experience of this type of detailed interviewing procedure spreads, research teams will discover members unable to meet the rating standards achieved by their fellows.

10. CONSISTENT BIAS BETWEEN RATERS

The experience in the short and concentrated 'learning week' suggests that raters can probably adopt the standards of others as they learn the PSE. In addition, it is necessary to examine the less artificially conducted field studies to see whether, under ordinary working conditions, members of research teams using the PSE regain their own individual levels of rating. It seems clear that they do not, for very little evidence of consistent differences, or bias, emerges from either the US–UK study (Kendell *et al.*, 1968) or from the study reported by Sartorius, Brooke and Lin (1970). Kendell and his colleagues carried out a three-way analysis of variance on their three-man reliability and repeatability study, which was capable of detecting consistent differences in level of rating between the three raters; in all analyses carried out, the mean squares for raters were not significant, implying that none of the raters had a detectable personal bias. The IPSS studies show that by some methods of analysis, no consistent bias could be found either between or within the various field centres, when the live interviews rated at each centre during the progress of the project were used. Separate analysis of the special reliability and teaching interviews, however, showed up a few individuals and one particular centre as having indentifiable tendencies to rate lower or higher than the rest, though not to an extent which could be regarded as invalidating the results.

In summary, it is concluded that so long as a properly designed programme of learning procedures and reliability studies is adhered to, the PSE can fulfil the aim of providing an acceptable degree of reliability and repeatability at all stages of the diagnostic process. However, there are circumstances which no general statements about reliability can cover and the results quoted in this chapter are compatible with occasional substantial differences between individual raters and between groups of raters in different centres. This problem will be discussed further in chapter 8.

6

THE CLASSIFICATION OF SYMPTOMS: THE CATEGO PROGRAM

The initial stages in the process of simulating the way a clinical diagnosis is made have now been described. Chapter 2 indicates how it is possible to standardise the collection of data. Chapters 3 and 4 describe the initial stages of data-reduction according to a clinical plan, and chapter 5 demonstrates that these procedures can be carried out reliably. Once the PSE ratings are made, the rest of the classification process should be automatic, with no room for further personal judgement apart from the specification of rules. These instructions are incorporated in a computer program known as Catego which will be described in this chapter. The program was written by Mrs Cynthia Taylor of the MRC Computer Services Centre (for the IPSS) and Miss Jane Gourlay (for the US–UK Project).

The complete program consists of ten stages, of which the first eight are concerned with reducing some 500 PSE items to at most six 'descriptive categories'. Patients are usually allocated only two or three of these but it is possible for a patient to be given all six. In stage 9, this material is concentrated even further so that each patient can be placed into one unique 'descriptive group'. Stage 10 deals with clinical data from the history of present and previous episodes and with possible aetiological factors such as heavy drinking, amphetamine abuse, the presence of organic disease, etc. Table 6.1 summarises the various stages in the program.

STAGE 1. DERIVATION OF SYMPTOMS

This has already been described in detail in chapter 3. PSE items are sorted into small groups, each representing one symptom. The ratings on each group of items are summed and, if the score reaches a threshold point (detailed for the MRC eighth edition in appendix 3.1) the symptom is said to be present.

Scores on delusional symptoms which are based only on ratings of (1) are differentiated by an asterisk, which singles them out for special treatment later in the program. In the ninth edition, the symptoms are directly rated and combination of items is therefore unnecessary.

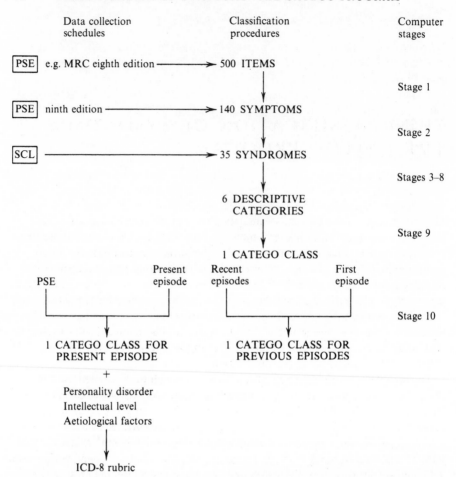

Figure 6.1. Stages of data collection and classification.

STATE 2. DERIVATION OF SYNDROMES

This has been described in detail in chapter 4. Only the first thirty-five syndromes in the syndrome check list presented in appendix 4.1 are used at present; in fact the classification would be very little different if only the first twenty-five were used. This is because the more important syndromes from a diagnostic point of view have low ordinal numbers. The principles by which syndromes are derived from symptoms are given in appendix 4.1. The computer prints out a list of syndromes, certainties and scores (the sum of constituent symptom scores), and the ratings on the constituent symptoms are shown for each syndrome.

STAGE 3. COMBINATION OF SYNDROMES 1–11

The next six stages of the computer program (stages 3–8) incorporate rules for the further combination of the syndromes in order to produce a number of descriptive categories. One patient may be allocated up to six of these, each with an appropriate degree of certainty, although usually only two or three are used. A patient allocated six categories would have shown an extremely mixed clinical picture, different elements of which would allow designation as schizophrenic, manic, depressed, anxious, hysterical and obsessional. Usually one of these categories would be more 'certain' than the others. The depressive category might be psychotic or non-psychotic. If no schizophrenic, manic or psychotic depressive category was allocated, a category of 'other psychosis' might be used. If no anxious, obsessional or non-psychotic depressive category was allocated, a category of 'other condition' might be used. If none of these categories could be allocated, the category 'no abnormality' would be used.

Due to the fact that the PSE schedule covers all the phenomena commonly encountered in the functional psychoses and neuroses, and there are obligatory questions in each area, it is quite common to find that a patient has several different types of symptomatology. From a descriptive point of view, the list of categories, with their degrees of certainty, is probably the most useful summary of PSE material. Although not as comprehensive as a list of syndromes, it still indicates the range of symptomatology present in a fairly concise way, without the rigidity imposed by having to place each patient into only one group.

In stage 3 certain syndromes (nos. 1–11) are used which, if they were present by themselves, would immediately suggest one particular diagnosis. Each such syndrome is converted directly into a 'potential category'. There may be several such potential categories, each suggesting a particular variety of schizophrenia, or depression or anxiety, in the same patient, but this overlapping is dealt with at a later stage. Thus (NS), (CS), (IS), (RS), (AF) are all potentially schizophrenic syndromes; (DD) and (SD) are potentially depressive; (GA) and (SA) are potentially representative of anxiety states; while (ON) and (HT) are the only potential representatives of obsessional neurosis and hysteria. Each of these eleven syndromes, if present, is therefore converted into a potential category, with the degree of certainty of the original syndrome. Certain syndromes are combined together to form further potential categories which are stored for later use.

The detailed rules for stage 3 are as follows:

3.1   *If syndromes (1)–(11) are not present, proceed to stage 4.*

3.2   *Combine certain syndromes to produce potential categories as follows:* *

3.2.1   (CS)+(OV)   ⟶   ECS

* The convention used to distinguish syndromes, categories and classes is as follows: syndrome 1, (NS); potential or descriptive category 1, NS; Catego class 1, *NS*.

3.2.2 (CS)+(SL) $\longrightarrow$ RCS
3.2.3 ECS+RCS $\longrightarrow$ MCS
3.2.4 (DD)+(SD) $\longrightarrow$ PD
3.2.5 PD or (DD)+SL $\longrightarrow$ RPD
3.2.6 PD or (DD)+AG $\longrightarrow$ APD
3.2.7 RPD+APD $\longrightarrow$ MPD
3.2.8 (DD) alone $\longrightarrow$ DD
3.2.9 (SD)+(SL) $\longrightarrow$ RSD ⎫
3.2.10 (SD)+(AG) $\longrightarrow$ ASD ⎪
3.2.11 (SD)+(TE) $\longrightarrow$ TSD ⎬   (If R and L, R > L
3.2.12 (SD)+(LE) $\longrightarrow$ LSD ⎪   If A and T, A > T)
3.2.13 ASD+RSD $\longrightarrow$ MSD ⎪
3.2.14 TSD+LSD $\longrightarrow$ TSD ⎭
3.2.15 (SA)+(GA) $\longrightarrow$ SA

3.3 *The certainty of syndrome (1)–(11) becomes the certainty of the potential categories, e.g.:*

   (DD++)+(AD?) = PD++
   (SD?)+(LE+) = LSD?

3.4 *When* (DD) *and* (SD) *are combined to produce PD,* (SD) *cannot be used again,* e.g. to produce RSD. PD may, however, be recombined, e.g. to produce RPD.

3.5 *Any syndrome* (1)–(11) *which has not been combined should be retained unchanged as a potential category.* Syndrome (AF) → SS.

3.6 *Combined syndromes and residual single syndromes are called potential categories.* Those so far derived are as follows:

   CS $\longrightarrow$ ECS, RCS, MCS
   DD $\longrightarrow$ PD, RPD, APD, MPD
   SD $\longrightarrow$ ASD, TSD, RSD, LSD, MSD
   GA $\longrightarrow$ SA
   NS
   IS
   RS
   ON
   HT
   SS

3.7 (OV) *and* (SL) *may be re-used in stage 4*, even if already used in stage 3. Any other syndrome used in stage 3 (i.e. converted into a potential category) should be discarded.

STAGE 4. COMBINATION OF SYNDROMES

In stage 4, syndromes 12–21 are considered for combination. These syndromes are diagnostically relevant but they do not, in themselves, suggest one particular diagnosis. Thus the delusional syndromes (PE) or (RE) or (GR) or (SF) may occur in several different psychotic conditions and their diagnostic significance depends upon the context of other syndromes. Once the syndromes are considered in twos, threes, fours or fives, however, the diagnostic problems usually become clearer, since only certain combinations are likely. However, *any* combination can theoretically occur (and, in fact, all combinations do sometimes occur in practice) and all must therefore be provided for. It is not feasible to allocate a potential category to every possible combination of ten syndromes, any number of which might be present. The method adopted has the merit of simplicity and it does take account, in a rough and ready way, both of clinical judgements concerning the potential diagnostic value of pairs of syndromes, and of the overall context of other syndromes present.

If more than five syndromes 12–21 are present, only the first five are considered (the order is given by the syndrome list, appendix 4.1). Syndromes with a query degree of certainty are omitted. (If *only* query syndromes are present the potential category is UP?.) (HM?) is an exception to this rule however. If only one or two syndromes are present, one or more potential categories are allocated, together with a degree of certainty. If three, four or five syndromes 12–21 are present, each pair is considered separately and rules are laid down for adding the resulting potential categories and certainties together and deciding upon a final one or two potential categories. The details are given in table 6.1.

Although this procedure may appear complex, every step in the procedure is precisely laid down so that a computer can follow it, and there is no possibility that different rules will be applied to different cases. The diagnostic process as followed by clinician consists of similar logical sequences. The difference is that the clinician can easily follow slightly different rules each time since the possibilities for variation are endless. The computer never varies if it is working correctly.

At the end of stage 4 every patient with one or more syndromes (12–21) has been allocated one or two potential categories each with a degree of certainty.

The detailed rules for stage 4 are as follows:

4.1   *If no syndromes 1–21, proceed to stage 7.*

4.2   *If no syndromes 12–21, proceed to stage 5.*

4.3   *Omit all ?syndromes (i.e. 14–19)* from consideration at this stage. Consider them in stage 7.

4.4   *If only one syndrome 12–21 is present*, derive the potential category and certainty from the last column of table 6.1

Table 6.1. *Combination of syndromes 12–21*

	12 (HM)	13 (AH)	14 (PE)	15 (RE)	16 (GR)	17 (SF)	18 (SH)	19 (OH)	20 (OV)	21 (SL)	Nil
12 (HM)	–	DS?	MN+ DP?	MN+	MN+	MN+ DP?	MN+ DP?	MN+	EMN+	MN? AP?	HM
13 (AH)		–	DS+	DS+	DS+	DS+	DS+	DS+	DS+	If combined DS+AP? If alone; DS?	DS
14 (PE)			–	DP? AP?	DP+ MN?	DP+	DP+ MN?	DP+ AP?	DP? MN?	DP? AP?	DP AP
15 (RE)				–	MN+ DP?	DP+	DP+ MN?	DP? AP?	DP? MN?	DP? AP?	DP AP
16 (GR)					–	DP+ MN?	DP? MN?	DP? MN?	MN+	MN? DP?	DP MN
17 (SF)						–	DP?	DP?	DP? MN?	DP?	DP
18 (SH)							–	DP? AP?	DP? AP?	DP? AP?	DP AP
19 (OH)								–	MN?	AP+	AP
20 (OV)									–	MN? AP?	–
21 (SL)										–	–

Combined degree of certainty

No. of syndromes	++	+	?	0
3	6	4, 5	2, 3	1
4	10+	7–9	4–6	1–3
5	17+	12–16	6–11	1–5

e.g. (GR++) $\longrightarrow$ DP?, MN?

   (GR+) $\longrightarrow$ DP?, MN?

The used syndrome is discarded.

(See, however, 4.5.2, if HM or MN are derived.)

4.5   *If only two syndromes 12–21 are present*, derive the potential category from the appropriate cell of table 6.1.

4.5.1   Ignore the certainty attached to the syndromes being combined.

4.5.2.   If no symptom 44 or 84 (list I)*

$$HM+ \longrightarrow Discard$$
$$MN+ \longrightarrow MN?$$
$$MN? \longrightarrow Discard$$
$$(e.g. \; DP?, MN+ \longrightarrow DP?, MN?$$
$$DP+, MN+ \longrightarrow DP+, MN?$$
$$DP?, MN? \longrightarrow DP?$$
$$DP+, MN? \longrightarrow DP+$$
$$MN?, AP? \longrightarrow AP?)$$

4.5.3   The two used syndromes are dropped from the program.

4.6   *If only three syndromes 12–21 are present*, derive the potential categories for each pair together with the certainties, according to the instructions given under 4.5 above.

Example 1: (AH+)+(PE++)+(SL+)
$$(AH+)+(PE++) \longrightarrow DS+$$
$$(AH+)+(SL+) \longrightarrow DS+, AP?$$
$$(PE++)+(SL+) \longrightarrow DP?, AP?$$

Example 2: (HM?)+(GR+)+(OV+)
$$(HM?)+(GR+) \longrightarrow MN?$$
$$(GR+)+(OV+) \longrightarrow MN+$$
$$(MN?)+OV+) \longrightarrow EMN?$$

4.6.1   If DP and DS are both potential categories, DP = DS.

4.6.2   If MN and EMN are present together, count both as MN.

4.6.3   Score the derived certainties as follows:
$$(+) = 2$$
$$(?) = 1$$

4.6.4   Sum the numerical equivalents of the certainties of each type of potential category.

4.6.5   Derive the new certainties as follows: $(6 = ++), (4, 5 = +), (2, 3 = ?), (1 = 0)$.

Example 1: DS+, DS+, DP? $\longrightarrow$ DS5 $\longrightarrow$ DS+
AP?, AP? $\longrightarrow$ AP2 $\longrightarrow$ AP?
Example 2: MN?, MN+, EMN? $\longrightarrow$ MN4 $\longrightarrow$ MN+

---

* This is automatically taken care of in the syndrome check list using list II symptoms (appendix 4.1).

4.6.6   If no symptom 44 or 84 (list I): see 4.5.2.

4.6.7   The three used syndromes are dropped from the program.

4.7   *If only four syndromes 12–21 are present*, use a similar procedure to that described under (4.6) above, but rescore as follows: $(10+ = ++)$, $(7-9 = +)$, $(4-6 = ?)$, $(1-3 = 0)$.

4.8   *If only five syndromes 12–21 are present*, use a similar procedure to that described under (4.6) above, but rescore as follows: $(17+ = ++)$, $(12-16 = +)$, $(6-11 = ?)$, $(1-5 = 0)$.

4.9   Discard the sixth and any subsequent syndrome 12–21, using the numerical order to judge precedence.

STAGE 5. COMBINATION OF POTENTIAL CATEGORIES SO FAR DERIVED

Stage 5 is a brief one, intended to tidy up any affective psychotic potential categories so far derived. DD or PD may have been derived from stage 3 and AP from stage 4, but only one category of this type goes forward.

The rules are as follows:

5.1.1   PD+AP?, + $\longrightarrow$ Increase PD by one degree

5.1.2   DD+AP?, + $\longrightarrow$ PD+

5.1.3   DD alone (no SD) $\longrightarrow$ AP with same certainty as originally

STAGE 6. DERIVATION OF 'S'-TYPE PSYCHOTIC CATEGORIES

A similar tidying up operation is carried out in stage 6 for any 'schizophrenic' potential categories so far derived. Ideally, only one category should remain at the end of this stage, though this cannot entirely be realised. If any categories NS, DS, (AH) are present together only the one with the highest rank order is retained. Similarly with the series CS, RS, IS, UP, SS. If one category from either of these series, or from both, is retained, the resulting category is derived from table 6.2. If category DP is also present, combination is delayed until stage 9.

The rules are as follows:

6.1   *If no 'S' potential categories* (table 6.2) $\longrightarrow$ Stage 7

6.2.1   If NS and DS together: increase certainty by one degree of certainty:

    e.g.   NS?+DS+ $\longrightarrow$ NS+
            NS++DS? $\longrightarrow$ NS++
            Discard DS when combined.

Table 6.2. *Combination of S-type potential categories*

	NS	DS	DP	CS	RS	IS	SS	Nil
NS	–	NS*	NS, DP†	CNS	NS	NS	NS	NS
DS		–	–	CDS	DS	DS	DS	DS
DP			–	CS, DP†	DP	DP	DP	DP

* Increase certainty of NS by one degree.
† Use certainty of constituent potential categories.

6.2.2   If no potential category from CS, RS, IS, SS series: and NS or DS are present without DP: convert to category as in right-hand column of table 6.2.

6.3.1   If CS, RS, IS, SS:
Use only the one with highest rank (in this order), irrespective of degree of certainty. Discard the others.

      e.g.   CS+, IS?, SS++ $\longrightarrow$ CS+
            IS?, SS+ $\longrightarrow$ IS?

6.3.2   If no potential category from NS, DS, DP series, convert to category as in right-hand column of table 6.2.

6.4   *If one potential category from the series* NS, DS, DP *and another from the series* CS, RS, IS, SS: select category from appropriate cell of table 6.2.

6.5   *If* DP *present:* enter table 6.2
      i.e.   if present alone $\longrightarrow$ DP
         if with another PC or category from 6.2.2, 6.3.2 or 6.4
           $\longrightarrow$ $\begin{array}{l} \text{NS, DP} \\ \text{CS, DP} \end{array}$ combine these in stage 9
         but RS, DP $\longrightarrow$ DP

STAGE 7. SYNDROME 22(NP) AND CATEGORY UP

In stages 5 and 6, categories NS, DS, DP, CS, RS, MN and PD (with their derivatives such as ECS, RPD etc.) have been derived. If any one of these is present, (NP) or UP are discarded. If partial delusions are present as the only delusional contribution, the category DP? is allocated. If UP or (NP) are present without any of these categories, certain rules are applied to produce further categories.

These are detailed as follows:

7.1   *If* NS, DS, DP, CS, RS, MN, PD, AP, HM *are so far derived:* discard (NP).

7.2   *Partial delusions only* (syndromes 14–17) ⟶ DP? and discard (NP).

7.3.1   UP+(NP) ⟶ UP with extra degree of certainty

7.3.2   (NP)+SS ⟶ UP?
         UP+SS   ⟶ UP

7.3.3   (NP) alone ⟶ UP?

7.4   SH? *or* OH? *only* ⟶ UP?

7.5   *Discard used or combined syndromes and potential categories.*

STAGE 8. PRINT OUT OF DESCRIPTIVE CATEGORIES

All the categories so far derived are printed out (see table 6.3). Categories 1–12 are known as S-type, since they are obviously related to schizophrenia. Categories 13,

Table 6.3. *List of categories printed out in stage 8*

1 NS		13 MN M-type		25 SD		38 ED	
2 CS		14 PD	D-type	26 SA		39 AH	
3 DS		15 AP		27 GA		40 OV	
4 DP		16 UP	U-type	28 ON		41 SL	
5 RS		17 XP		29 XN		42 DD	
6 SS	S-type	18 EMN	M-type	30 ASD	N-type	43 IS	Tem-
7 ECS		19 DMN		31 TSD		44 HT	porary
8 RCS		20 RPD		32 RSD		45 DE	cate-
9 MCS		21 APD	D-type	33 LSD		Synd. 23	gories
10 CNS		22 MPD		34 MSD		46 AG	
11 CDS		23 MAP	M-type	35 MAN		Synd. 25	
12 IDS		24 HM		36 XX		47 NG	
				37 NO		Synd. 26	
						48 Synds. 28–35	

Each category is present in one of three degrees of certainty (?, +, ++).

Categories 1–12 = S-type
Categories 13, 18, 19, 23, 24 = M-type ⎫
Categories 14, 15, 20, 21, 22 = D-type ⎬ P-type
Categories 16, 17 = U-type   ⎭

Categories 25–36   N-type

18, 19 and 24 are M (manic)-type. Categories 14, 15, 20, 21, 22 are D (psychotic depressive)-type. Category 16 is U (non-specific psychosis)-type.

All the above categories are P (psychotic)-type. Categories 25–36 are N (neurotic)-type, including depressive, anxiety, obsessional and residual categories. There are also some temporary categories carried over for action in later stages.

It is possible for one patient with a particularly complex clinical picture to be allocated a category from the 'S' series, one from the 'D' series (which might be psychotic or not), one from the 'M' series, one from the 'anxiety' series and one from the 'obsessional' series. Each category has its own degree of certainty. Thus the clinical picture is summarised under these five headings before any attempt is made to fit the patient into only one class. Stage 8 therefore constitutes an informative clinical description of each patient, since the information available in the eighth edition is reduced from 500 items to 5, but the variety which may be present in the clinical picture is to a reasonable extent preserved.

STAGE 9. DERIVATION OF CATEGO CLASSES

Although the descriptive categories are very useful clinically, because they represent the range of symptoms present, each variety with its degree of certainty, it is necessary to allocate each patient to only one class (perhaps with one alternative class in certain cases) if a diagnosis is eventually to be made. This reduction necessarily involves a loss of information and therefore the chief problem to be solved in stage 9 of the Catego program lies in deciding what should be omitted. The main priorities are laid down by the degrees of certainty of each category but categories are also ranked in a hierarchy. Eventually, each patient is allocated to one of fifty classes, which leaves plenty of scope for expressing any diversity in the symptomatology, but there has to be a further reduction, to only sixteen classes, in order to prepare for the next stage.

Single P-categories are converted directly into the appropriate class but *UP* and *SS* are regarded as borderline and another class is also allocated on the basis of any non-psychotic symptoms present. These are the only exceptions to the rule that one patient is allocated to one class.

If more than one P-category is present, detailed rules are laid down showing which takes priority. Non-psychotic categories are discarded. Rank in the hierarchy and degree of certainty are both taken into account. Schizophrenic categories have a higher ranking than manic or depressive or uncertain. If the manic depressive categories have a high degree of certainty, however, a schizo-affective class can be used. Specific rules are laid down to deal with situations in which both catatonic *and* psychotic depressive categories, or both non-nuclear delusional *and* manic categories are present. All possible combinations are covered. Inevitably, all decisions are quite arbitrary and a clinician might arrive at some other judgement by taking extra information into account. This, the computer is not allowed to do.

Table 6.4. *Catego III: Catego classes coding key*

x 50		x 16	x 9		x 50		x 16	x 9	
01	NS+	01	2	S+	26	CSMN	05	1	O+
02	NS?	01	2	S+	27	MNRS	08	5	M+
03	DS+	01	2	S+	28	RSMN	05	1	O+
04	DS?	14	2	S?	29	NSPD, DSPD	04	2	S+
05	DP+	02	7	P+	30	DPPD	15	7	P+
06	DP?	03	7	P?	31	DP? AP?	03	7	P?
07	CS	05	1	O+	32	PDRS	07	4	D?
08	RS+	05	1	O?	33	RSPD	05	1	O+
09	RS?	10	1	O?	34	CSPD	05	1	O+
10	SS	10	1	O?	35	XP	10	1	O?
11	PD+	06	4	D+	36	ON+	16	8	B+
12	PD?	07	4	D?	37	ON?	16	8	B?
13	MN+	08	5	M+	38	ND+	12	9	N+
14	MN?	09	5	M?	39	MN?	12	9	N?
15	HM+	11	5	M+	40	SD+	12	9	N+
16	-	-	-	-	41	SD?	12	9	N?
17	UP+	10	1	O?	42	RD+	13	4	R+
18	UP?	10	1	O?	43	RD?	12	9	N?
19	AP+	07	4	D?	44	AN+	16	8	A+
20	AP?	07	4	D?	45	AN?	16	8	A?
21	MAP+	08	5	M+	46	PN+	16	8	A+
22	NSMN, DSMN	04	2	S+	47	PN?	16	8	A?
23	DPMN	15	7	P+	48	HT	16	8	H
24	-	-	-	-	49	XN	16	8	X
25	MNCS	08	5	M+	50	NO	00	0	-
					00	Ep, 44	00	0	

If no psychotic categories are present, the non-psychotic categories are considered and, by the application of similar decisions based on rank in the hierarchy and degree of certainty, each patient is allocated to one non-psychotic class. Patients can be allocated to classes representing 'retarded depression', 'neurotic depression', 'obsessional neurosis', 'phobic anxiety', 'general anxiety state' or 'hysteria'. If the patient shows only a non-specific syndrome such as worrying or irritability, the class allocated is 'other neurosis'. Finally, there is a class, 'no abnormality', to cover patients for whom no syndrome at all has been rated at present. The full list of fifty classes is given in table 6.4.

The detailed rules are as follows:

9.1 *Single psychotic categories*

9.1.1 Consider only second two letters of categories, except for EMN and the combinations of SD which are dealt with specifically under later headings.

9.1.2   If only U-type categories 6 SS; 16 UP; also allocate a class based on remaining categories. (If SS+HM, discard SS.) (See also 9.2.5.)

9.1.3   Convert single P-type and U-type categories to equivalent classes as follows:

1	*NS*+, ++	11	*PD*+, ++
2	*NS*?	12	*PD*?
3	*DS*+, ++	13	*MN*+, ++
4	*DS*?	14	*MN*?
5	*DP*+, ++	15	*HM*+, ++
6	*DP*?	16	*HM*?
7	*CS*+, ++	17	*UP*+, ++
8	*RS*+, ++	18	*UP*?
9	*RS*?	19	*AP*+, ++
10	*SS*+, ++	20	*AP*?

9.2   >*1 psychotic category (1-24)*

9.2.1   Discard 6, SS or 16, UP categories.

9.2.2   If 24, HM and another P-category are present, HM ⟶ MN.

9.2.3   If 13, MN and 14, PD (or 15, AP) only (no schizophrenic categories):

HM, MN > PD ⟶ *MN* (13 or 14)

PD, AP > HM, MN ⟶ *PD* (11) or *AP* (19)

using whichever degree of certainty is greater.

9.2.4   If S-category+(M-category+D-category) present together, discard the M-category or D-category with lesser degree of certainty. If the M-category and D-category are equal in degree of certainty use M-category only.

9.2.5   RS+ with MN, PD, AP ⟶ Ignore RS

RS+ alone ⟶ 9, *RS*? = BP category, i.e. double grouping

RS++ and MN, PD, AP ⟶ 28, *RS/MN*

33, *RS/PD*

RS++ and DP or DP/MN ⟶ Ignore RS++

RS++ alone ⟶ 8, *RS*+

9.2.6   If NS and DP or CS and DP are present together, with an M-category or D-category, first combine DP and the M- or D-category according to the rules in 9.3.5 and 9.4.5. Then add NS or CS according to the special notes.

9.2.7   If no M- or D-category

NS:DP   ⟶ NS+ or NS?

CS > DP   ⟶ 7, *CS*

DP > CS   ⟶ 5, *DP*+

9.3 *Combine S-category and M-category as follows:*

9.3.1 *NS:MN*   MN > NS $\longrightarrow$ 22, *NS/MN*
               NS = > MN $\longrightarrow$ 1, *NS+* or 2, *NS?*

9.3.2 *NS:EMN* Discard EMN.

9.3.3 *DS:MN*   MN = > DS $\longrightarrow$ 22, *DS/MN*
               DS > MN $\longrightarrow$ 3, *DS+*

9.3.4 *DS:EMN* Discard EMN.

9.3.5 *DP:MN*

9.3.5.1   MN = > DP $\longrightarrow$ 13, *MN+* or 14, *MN?*
               DP > MN $\longrightarrow$ 23, *DP/MN*

9.3.5.2 *If NS as well as DP:MN*
          NS:MN as in 9.3.1
          NS:DP $\longrightarrow$ 1, *NS+* or 2, *NS?*
          NS:DP/MN $\longrightarrow$ 1, *NS+* or 2, *NS?*

9.3.5.3 *If CS as well as DP:MN*
          CS:MN as in 9.3.7 below
          CS > DP $\longrightarrow$ 7, *CS*
          DP = > CS $\longrightarrow$ 5, *DP+*
          CS:DP/MN $\longrightarrow$ 23, *DP/MN*

9.3.6 *DP:EMN* This combination should not occur.

9.3.7 *CS:MN*
          MN > CS $\longrightarrow$ 25, *MN/CS*
          MN = CS $\longrightarrow$ 26, *CS/MN*
          CS > MN $\longrightarrow$ 7, *CS*

9.3.8 *CS:EMN*
          EMN > CS $\longrightarrow$ 26, *CS/MN*
          CS = > EMN $\longrightarrow$ 7, *CS*

9.3.9 *RS:EMN* As for 9.3.9, RS:MN.

9.4 *Combine S-category and D-category as follows:*

9.4.1 *NS:PD*
          PD > NS $\longrightarrow$ 29, *NS/PD*
          NS = > PD $\longrightarrow$ 1, *NS+* or 2, *NS?*

9.4.2 *NS:AP* Discard AP.

9.4.3 *DS:PD*
          PD = > DS $\longrightarrow$ 29, *PS/PD*
          DS > PD $\longrightarrow$ 3, *DS+*

9.4.4 *DS:AP* Discard AP.

9.4.5   *DP:PD*

9.4.5.1   PD = > DP ⟶ 11, *PD*+ or 12, *PD*?
                 DP > PD   ⟶ 30, *DP/PD*

9.4.5.2   *If NS as well as DP:PD*
          NS : PD as in 9.4.1 above
          NS : DP   ⟶ 1, *NS*+ or 2, *NS*?
          NS : DP/PD ⟶ 1, *NS*+ or 2, *NS*?

9.4.5.3   *If CS as well as DP:PD*
          CS : PD as in 9.4.9 below
          CS > DP   ⟶ 7, *CS*
          DP = > CS ⟶ 5, *DP*+
          CS : DP/PD ⟶ 30, *DP/PD*

9.4.6   *DP: AP* only (no NS, CS or RS)

9.4.6.1   DP > AP   ⟶ 5, *DP*+
                 AP = > DP ⟶ 31, *DP/AP*?

9.4.6.2   If DP : AP *and* NS, CS
          First combine DP, AP as in 9.4.6.1
          If ⟶ DP+ combine according to established rules
          If ⟶ DP?, AP?, treat as DP? and combine according to
          established rules

9.4.7   *CS:PD*
                 PD > CS   ⟶ 11, *PD*+
                 CS = > PD ⟶ 34, *CS/PD*

9.4.8   *CS:AP*   All combinations ⟶ 7, *CS*+

(BP) *category*

9.5   If the only P-categories are U-type (i.e. 9, RS?; 6, SS; 16, UP) allocate another
      group in the same way as if no P-categories were present, and print out both
      in 9.12.

9.6   *Derivation of non-psychotic groups*

9.6.1   ON++ (and one item rated 2) ⟶ 36, *ON*+
        (Consider ON+ and ON? and other ON++ at 9.7.)

9.6.2   SD?, +, ++ with (SL), AG, ED, SA, GA:

9.6.2.1   SD+ (SL) ⟶ 42, *RD*+ or 43, *RD*?
          SD+ (AG) ⟶ 42, *RD*+ or 43, *RD*?
          depending on certainty of SD
          i.e. syndromes 21, (SL) and 25 (AG) automatically convert SD to *RD*
          with certainty of SD.

9.6.2.2   Combine categories SD and ED as follows:

	EDO	ED+	ED++
SD?	SD?	RD?	RD++
SD+	SD+	RD+	RD++
SD++	SD++	RD+	RD++

If SA or GA are O or ?, take group from appropriate cell in table
(RD++ $\longrightarrow$ 42, *RD*+   SD++ $\longrightarrow$ 40, *SD*+)
If SA or GA are + or ++,   RD++ $\longrightarrow$ 42, *RD*+
                            RD+ $\longrightarrow$ 40, *SD*+
                            RD? $\longrightarrow$ 41, *SD*?
                            SD $\longrightarrow$ 9.6.2.3

9.6.2.3   Combine SD, and GA or SA (whichever has higher certainty; if GA = SA, drop GA), as follows:

	GA/SA+	GA/SA++
SD?	AN/PN+	AN/PN+
SD+	ND+	AN/PN+
SD++	ND+	ND+
	(38, *ND*+	39, *ND*?)

9.6.3   *If* GA *or* SA, *but no* SD:
          GA > SA $\dashrightarrow$ 44, *AN*+ or 45, *AN*?
          SA = > GA $\longrightarrow$ }
          SA = GA $\longrightarrow$ } 46, *PN*+ or 47, *PN*?

9.7   *If no* SD, *or* GA:SA, *but* ON+ *or* ?:
          ON+ or ? $\longrightarrow$ 36, *ON*+ or 37, *ON*?

9.8   *If no* GA:SA, SD *or* ON, *but* HT:
          HT $\longrightarrow$ 48, *HT*

9.9   *If no* UP, SS, RS, SD, GA:SA, ON *or* HT, *but one of* SD, OV, DE, AG *or* NG:
          $\longrightarrow$ 35, *XP*

9.10 *If none of these (9.9), but* ED *or syndromes 28–35:*
          $\longrightarrow$ 49, *XN*

9.11 *If none of these (9.10):*
          $\longrightarrow$ 50, *NO*

9.12 Print out Catego class for PSE. Give number of 50-class, 16-class, and 9-class classification (table 6.4).

STAGE 10. COMBINATION OF CATEGO CLASSES FOR PRESENT AND PREVIOUS EPISODES

So far, we have been considering data derived only from the PSE which, by the time stage 9 has been reached, are sifted and combined so that the clinical picture is allocated to one descriptive class. Clearly, a similar process can be applied to SCL data derived from records or other information concerning the present episode of illness, so that two Catego classes can be derived, one from the PSE and one from the SCL of the present episode. Table 6.5 shows how the two classes (in the 16-class form) can be combined to give one overall class.

Table 6.5. *Combination of Catego classes (x16)*

	1	2	3	4	5	6	7	8	9	10	11	12	13	14	15	16
1	1	1	1	1	1	4	1	4	1	1	1	1	1	1	1	1
2		2	2	4	2	15	2	15	2	2	15	2	2	1	2	2
3			3	4	5	6	3	8	3	3	11	3	3	14	15	3
4				4	4	4	4	4	4	4	4	4	4	1	4	4
5					5	6	5	8	5	5	5	5	5	14	15	5
6						6	6	8	8	6	8	6	6	7	7	6
7							7	8	9	7	8	7	6	4	15	7
8								8	8	8	8	8	8	9	9	8
9									9	9	8	9	9	4	15	9
10										10	11	10,12	10,13	14	15	10,16
11											11	12	13	4	9	11
12												12	12	14	15	12
13													13	14	15	12
14														14	14	14
15															15	15
16																16

Apart from clear-cut changes such as loss of memory and changes in level of consciousness, the clinical 'present state' in most psychiatric conditions is covered by the symptoms rated in the PSE. Thus the symptomatic psychoses, or a depressive state secondary to personality disorder or alcohol addiction, rarely show specific symptoms; the diagnosis is made on the clinician's judgement of aetiology. In order to systematise these judgements somewhat, an 'aetiology schedule' has been drawn up which is presented in appendix 6.1. This is not intended as more than a guide to clinicians and research workers who wish to systematise their diagnostic judgements when deciding what patients to admit to a series, or how to describe a group of patients for clinical purposes. It has not yet been used in a large-scale study and no further claims can be made for it at the moment.

If no organic aetiology is thought to be present and the disorder, if non-psychotic,

Table 6.6. *Coding key for ICD, eighth edition diagnosis*

		x 36	x 18	x 9
295.0	Simple schizophrenia	01	01	1
295.1	Hebephrenic s.	02	02	2
295.2	Catatonic s.	03	03	1
295.3	Paranoid s.	04	04	2
295.4	Acute s.	05	05	2
295.5	Latent s.	06	06	1
295.6	Residual s.	07	07	1
295.7	Schizo-affective ps.	08	08	2
295.8	Other schizophrenic ps.	09	09	3
295.9	Schizophrenia NOS	10	10	3
296.0	Involutional melancholia	11	11	4
296.1	Mania	12	12	5
296.2	Psychotic depression	13	11	4
296.3	Manic-depressive psychosis	14	12	5
296.8	Other affective psychosis	15	13	6
296.9	Affective psychosis NOS	16	13	6
297.0	Paranoia	17	14	7
297.1	Involutional paraphrenia	18	14	7
297.9	Other paranoid psychosis	19	14	7
298.0	Reactive depressive psychosis	20	11	4
298.1	Reactive excitement	21	12	5
298.2	Reactive confusion	22	14	7
298.3	Reactive paranoid psychosis	23	14	7
298.9	Reactive psychosis NOS	24	14	7
299	Psychosis NOS	25	14	7
300.0–3 } 300.5–9	Neuroses	26	15	8
300.4	Depressive neurosis	27	16	9
310.0–9	Personality disorder	28	15	8
–	Psychogenic paranoid ps.	29	14	7
–	Acute paranoid ps.	30	14	7
–	Shift-like schizophrenia	31	09	3
–	Sluggish schizophrenia	32	06	1
–	Periodic schizophrenia	33	09	3
298.1	Hysterical psychosis	34	17	0
–	Puerperal psychosis	35	18	0
–	Organic conditions	36	18	0
–	No abnormality	00	00	0

Table 6.7. *Derivation of ICD diagnosis of organic aetiology*

Section 1 of aetiology schedule	Catego class S, P, O+, M, D PDG = Psychotic	Catego class O?, R, N, A, B, H, X PDG = Non-psychotic
Item		
1.1	290	309
1.2	292/3	309
1.3	294	309
1.4	299	309
1.5	304	304
1.6	291	303
1.7	294.4	No change
1.8	Class D $\longrightarrow$ 296.0	No change
	Class S or P $\longrightarrow$ 297.1	
	Class O+ or M $\longrightarrow$ No change	

is not thought to be secondary to personality abnormality, the 9-class grouping derived from table 6.4 is approximately equivalent to the 9-class diagnostic grouping shown in table 6.6. Class 8 can be further subdivided into anxiety or phobic state (class A; 300.0 and 300.2), obsessional neurosis (class B; 300.3), hysteria (class H; 300.1) and other neurosis (class X), while the aetiology schedule gives a judgement as to whether any neurotic condition is secondary to personality disorder. If some organic cause or influence is recorded in the aetiology schedule, the nearest ICS diagnosis can be read from the list in table 6.7. These final steps in reaching a diagnosis have not been programmed for the computer but they are very simple to apply. The main aim of the Catego procedure is not to reach an ICD diagnosis, since this classification itself needs much improvement. The main aim is to reach a categorisation by steps that are communicable and repeatable, so that the same procedure carried out in different parts of the world will yield groups that are in some specifiable sense comparable.

10.1   Derive descriptive groups for present episode (10.1.1), recent episodes (10.1.2) and first episode (10.1.3), using appropriate syndrome check lists.

10.2   Combine descriptive groups (x 16) for PSE and present episode from table 6.5.

10.3   Combine descriptive groups (x 16) for recent episodes and first episode from table 6.5.

N.B.   Ratings of personality disorder, intellectual level and aetiology may be derived from aetiology schedule (appendix 6.1). ICD-8 rubric may be derived from table 6.7 if organic aetiology present. If no organic aetiology, the Catego Diagnostic Group (x 9) in table 6.4 is compatible with the equivalent group (x 9) in table 6.6.

Having described the way in which such classes can be derived, it is next necessary to discover whether they do, in fact, bear any relationship to the diagnoses clinicians make in practice. Fortunately, two large international studies have been conducted in which psychiatrists of widely different backgrounds have used the PSE interview. It is therefore possible to subject the system to some fairly stiff preliminary tests. The results are examined in chapter 7.

APPENDIX 6.1

AETIOLOGY SCHEDULE

MRC Social Psychiatry Unit,
Institute of Psychiatry,
London S.E.5.

Project no.

Subject no.

Card no.

Episode number _____

Dates _____

The term aetiology is used broadly, to include factors modifying or obscuring the clinical picture during the episode being rated (e.g. cultural factors in a recent immigrant) as well as direct precipitants (e.g. amphetamine) and factors maintaining the illness. Rate as many factors in sections 1 and 2 as necessary.

    0 = Factor not present

    1 = Factor present: not modifying clinical picture and probably contributing very little to cause or precipitation

    2 = Factor present: modifying clinical picture and/or contributing to onset or maintenance of symptoms. Not the main cause or precipitant

    3 = Factor probably the main cause or precipitant of the episode of illness. Episode would probably not have occurred at this time without it (e.g. amphetamine psychosis, alcoholic hallucinosis)

    8 = Not known

    9 = Not applicable

1. ORGANIC FACTORS

1.0   If no such factors present, rate (0) here and proceed to 2.0

1.1   Senile or presenile dementia

1.2   Cerebral disease (arteriosclerosis, epilepsy, intracranial neoplasms, degenerative CNS disease, brain trauma, CNS syphilis and other infections, etc.)
Specify   ☐

1.3   Toxic factors acting on the brain other than above (endocrine, metabolic, nutritional, systemic infections, poison intoxication, etc.)
Specify   ☐

1.4   Perceptual or communication difficulty (blindness, deaf and dumb, aphasia etc.)
Specify   ☐

1.5   Drug abuse (not just overdose = 1.3)
Specify predominant drug   ☐

1.6   Alcohol abuse
Specify whether episodic or habitual excessive drinking or alcoholic addiction   ☐

1.7   Childbirth (onset within 4 weeks of delivery)   ☐

1.8   Menopause   ☐

2. SOCIAL OR PSYCHOLOGICAL FACTORS

2.0   If no such factors present, rate (0) here and proceed to 3.0   ☐

2.1   Adolescence   ☐

2.2   Member of special subcultural group   ☐

2.3   Recent immigration   ☐

2.4   Recent psychological or social conflicts, e.g. marital disharmony, separation, grief, employment problems, compensation, etc.   ☐

2.5   Educational backwardness or native language not English   ☐

2.6   Sexual deviation
      Specify

2.7   Other
      Specify

Specify example of any factor present:

3. PERSONALITY BEFORE FIRST ONSET

Rate the ICD characteristics listed on following scale: (only *one* category may be rated 2 or 1).

  See ICD glossary for definition.

  0 = Personality within normal limits (define broadly)
  1 = Personality definitely unusual and impairs patient's social adaptation, but not sufficient to make a main diagnosis of personality disorder
  2 = Personality markedly unusual – sufficient to make a main diagnosis of personality disorder. Catego classification of this episode is therefore secondary

3.0.0   No personality disorder, rate (0) here and cut-off

3.0   Paranoid   (301.0)

3.1   Affective   (301.1)

3.2   Schizoid   (301.2)

3.3   Explosive   (301.3)

3.4   Anankastic   (301.4)

3.5   Hysterical   (301.5)

3.6   Asthenic   (301.6)

3.7   Antisocial   (301.7)

3.8   Other, specify (301.8)   ☐

3.9   Unspecified   (301.9)   ☐

4. INTELLECTUAL LEVEL DURING EPISODE

(Rate only one category positively, 0 = No, 1 = Yes)

4.1   Ever ascertained as severely retarded   ☐

4.2   Ever attended ESN school   ☐

4.3   IQ < 80   ☐

4.4   IQ 81–100   ☐

4.5   IQ 101–115   ☐

4.6   IQ 116+   ☐

4.7   IQ not known. Probably below average   ☐

4.8   IQ not known. Probably average   ☐

4.9   IQ not known. Probably above average   ☐

If IQ tested, give dates, tests used and results: ☐

7

THE CATEGO CLASSES*

1. TWO LARGE-SCALE INTERNATIONAL PROJECTS IN WHICH THE PSE HAS BEEN USED

Data are available from two studies in which the PSE was used on a large scale; the US-UK Diagnostic Project and the WHO International Pilot Study of Schizophrenia (IPSS). The main publications of these studies should be consulted for details of aims, design, methods and results (Cooper *et al.*, 1972; WHO, 1973) and only a very brief account will be given here, in order to make clear the context of the results using the Catego procedure.

The US-UK Diagnostic Project had two main parts. In the first, two series of 250 patients aged 20–59, one admitted to Netherne Hospital, south of London, the other to Brooklyn State Hospital, New York, were examined using the seventh edition of the PSE and a specially constructed history schedule. A 'project diagnosis' was made using the ICD (eighth revision) and the English Glossary (GRO, 1968). The diagnoses made by the hospital clinicians were also recorded. In the second part of the study, 192 patients were drawn from the nine State hospitals covering New York City, and 174 from nine of the eighteen area hospitals covering Greater London; the age range was also 20–59 years. These patients were interviewed using the eighth edition of the PSE. Thus 866 patients were included in the two parts of the study. Of these, 688 were given diagnoses of schizophrenia, affective psychosis or neurosis, other neurosis or personality disorder.

Nine Centres took part in the International Pilot Study of Schizophrenia: Aarhus, Agra, Cali, Ibadan, London, Moscow, Taipei, Prague and Washington. Approximately 130 patients were assessed in each area, according to operational criteria designed to select only those probably suffering from one of the functional psychoses, except that about ten patients with neurotic depression were included from each Centre for purposes of comparison. In all, 1202 patients were included; each being interviewed using the WHO version of the eighth edition (translated into the

* This chapter is based largely upon data and experience obtained during (1) the International Pilot Study of Schizophrenia, a project sponsored by the World Health Organisation, the National Institute of Mental Health (United States), and the participating field research centres, and (2) the US–UK Diagnostic Project which was funded by NIMH and undertaken by Biometrics Research, New York State Department of Mental Hygiene, New York and the Institute of Psychiatry, London. A full list of all investigators and staff is presented in the acknowledgements.

appropriate languages) and being given a project diagnosis from the ICD. Historical and social data were also collected.

Certain changes were introduced into the Catego program following testing of the early versions on the first half of the IPSS series; these are detailed in chapter 11 of the first volume of the IPSS report.

A more important problem arising from the early testing was that items concerning auditory hallucinations in the seventh and eighth editions of the PSE were not sufficiently varied. The only discrimination allowed was between voices experienced as speaking about the patient and voices speaking to him, but this did not allow a differentiation of affectively-based or subculturally-based auditory hallucinations which was necessary for an accurate diagnosis. By consulting the examples of such ratings, written in the PSE schedules at the time of interview, it was usually possible to decide what kind of hallucinations were involved. In the IPSS series, auditory hallucinations were rated as present in ten cases with a project diagnosis of depressive psychosis (usually 296.2) and twelve with a project diagnosis of mania (296.1 or 296.3). This led to a Catego grouping in class S. All twenty-two had had the experience of hearing voices talking to them and four had also heard voices talking about them (in occasional single sentences; for example, 'He's a homosexual'). If the auditory hallucinations were excluded from the PSE input to the Catego program, the descriptive class allocated became concordant with the project diagnosis in all twenty-two cases. This change was therefore made.

In order to check that this procedure was valid, the narrative summaries of all the equivalent Netherne and UK patients from the US–UK series were rated blind, together with the next two cases with the same project diagnosis. In seven out of eight cases, affectively-based hallucinations were correctly identified, judged by the project diagnosis. In the other six cases where hallucinations were present, the concordant decision was made that they were not affectively based. The same modification was therefore made as in the IPSS material; in cases where the sole reason for a discrepancy between Catego class and project diagnosis was the presence of affectively based or subculturally based hallucinations, this rating was omitted from the PSE input.

The rating of hallucinations has been modified in the light of this experience and, in the ninth edition of the PSE, it is possible to rate affectively based and subculturally based hallucinations separately, so that this particular problem should not arise in future.

2. THE CLINICAL MEANING OF THE CATEGO CLASSES

It was shown in chapter 6 that PSE data could be combined, according to specified principles incorporated in a computer program, so as to allocate any individual to only one descriptive class. The complete system provides fifty classes, which allows fair scope for distinguishing patients with various types of mixed symptomatology.

For convenience of statistical treatment, however, these fifty classes need to be collapsed to only sixteen, or even fewer. The clinical meaning of these classes can be indicated by their relationship to the diagnoses made by clinicians (on the basis of all the information available, not just that contained in the PSE) and also by presenting syndrome and symptom profiles of the various classes.

Data from the US–UK and IPSS projects will mainly be used, but one further study, conducted by Binitie in Benin, mid-western Nigeria, will also be drawn upon because of its special clinical interest and because of its inclusion of a large number of patients diagnosed as 'anxiety states', which are hardly represented in the larger series.

In the first place, the relationship to clinical diagnoses of the Catego classes derived from PSE data alone will be considered and a comparison with an alternative means of predicting diagnosis (using Bayes' theorem) will also be presented. The PSE syndrome profiles of the collapsed Catego classes will then be examined. This will prepare the way for a consideration of the effects of adding data from the psychiatric history (PH).

3. COMPARISON OF CLINICAL DIAGNOSIS AND CLASSIFICATION BY CATEGO (PSE DATA ONLY)

In the first instance, a simple three-way classification into (i) schizophrenic and paranoid psychoses, (ii) manic psychoses and (iii) depressive psychoses and neuroses will be used. In terms of the International Classification of Diseases, these are very mixed bags indeed as can be seen from the following list:

Schizophrenic psychoses: 295.0–9, sluggish*, shift-like,* periodic* schizophrenia	S+, S?, O+, O?
Paranoid psychoses: 297.0, 297.0, 298.2, 298.3, 298.9, 299, psychogenic paranoid psychosis,† acute paranoid psychosis†	P+, P?
Manic psychoses: 296.1, 296.3, 298.1 (reactive excitement)	M+, M?
Depressive psychoses: 296.0, 296.2, 296.8, 296.9, 298.0	D+, D?, (R)
Depressive neuroses: 300.4	N, (R)
Other neuroses: 300.1–3, 5–9	A, B, H, X
Personality disorders: 301.1–9	–

* These diagnoses could be allotted to 295.8.
† These diagnoses are difficult to allot to an ICD rubric.

Table 7.1. *Diagnostic and Catego classes compared (IPSS series, PSE only)*

IPSS Project diagnosis	Catego class (PSE only)				
	S, O, P	M	D, R, N	Total	A, B, H, X
Schizophrenic and paranoid psychoses	720	61	86	867	11
Manic psychoses	12	62	3	77	2
Depressive psychoses and neuroses	34	6	135	175	1
Total	766	129	224	1119	14
Other neuroses and personality disorders	8	4	31	43	10
Other conditions	7	2	6	15	1

Neuroses other than depressive, personality disorders, addictions and organic conditions were fairly uncommon in the two series studied and, apart from non-depressive neuroses, they cannot be derived from PSE data alone. They are not therefore examined with the same attention as the others. Table 7.1 shows the degree of concordance between a crude three-way classification of clinical diagnoses with an equivalent grouping of Catego classes, using IPSS data.

There is, in fact, a very marked degree of association, so much so that 82% of cases are concordantly classified. Further details are given in table 7.2, from which it can be seen that there are 118 cases in uncertain classes (P?, O?, M?, D?) and 116 in classes R and N, representing the non-psychotic depressions. Clearly these classes could be readily changed by the addition of data from the history, since the PSE represents the clinical picture during a very brief period of time, whereas a clinical diagnosis is based upon all the information available to a clinician, including that gained from a study of the clinical history.

It is quite possible for the categorisation to be changed from several of the more certain classes (P+, O+, M+, D+) as well. Table 6.5 gives the rules for this. Only class S+ is unlikely to be changed, whatever historical data are added (with the exception of information about an organic aetiology).

It will therefore be wise to postpone a consideration of the degree of concordance between Catego classes and ICD diagnoses until data from the history have been taken into account. However the equivalent data from the US–UK project are first presented, in table 7.3, since they will be needed for comparison in the next section. The degree of condordance in a three-way table is very striking (80.7%).

Table 7.2. *Detailed diagnostic and Catego classes compared (IPSS series, PSE only)*

IPSS Project diagnosis	Catego class (PSE only)												Total	A, B, H, X
	S+	S?	P+	P?	O+	O?	M+	M?	D+	D?	R	N		
Schizophrenic psychoses	494	17	54	42	41	13	39	21	13	3	29	35	801	9
Paranoid psychoses	30	2	18	7	1	1	1	–	2	–	2	2	66	2
Manic psychoses	9	–	2	1	–	–	54	8	2	–	–	1	77	2
Depressive psychoses	8	1	5	10	1	–	2	2	29	2	24	22	106	–
Depressive neuroses	1	1	–	6	–	1	1	1	7	–	24	27	69	–
Total	542	21	79	66	43	15	97	32	53	5	79	87	1119	14
Other neuroses	2	–	1	1	2	1	3	–	1	–	4	21	36	8
Personality disorders	–	–	–	1	–	–	1	–	–	–	–	5	7	2
Other diagnoses	4	–	1	2	–	–	1	1	2	–	–	4	15	1

Table 7.3. *Diagnostic and Catego classes compared (US–UK series; PSE only)*

US–UK Project diagnosis	S, O, P	M	D, R, N	Total	A, B, H, X
Schizophrenic and paranoid psychoses	191	17	31	239	19
Manic psychoses	13	39	3	55	4
Depressive psychoses and neuroses	22	24	230	276	10
Total	226	80	264	570	33
Other neuroses and personality disorders	9	8	51	68	17

4. PREDICTION OF PROJECT DIAGNOSIS USING A BAYESIAN ANALYSIS OF PSE DATA

Given the symptom profile of each patient in a series, together with the psychiatric diagnosis in each case, it is possible to derive a set of probabilities which will allow the prediction of the most likely diagnosis using the PSE symptoms alone. This procedure, which is based upon Bayes' theorem, applies only to the series used to derive the set of probabilities; it would not necessarily apply to the same extent to any other series. The statistical analysis involves calculating the probability at which each symptom occurs in each diagnostic group and then cumulating the probabilities for the pattern of symptoms present in any particular case. It is necessary to assume that the symptoms occur independently within any disease group (Birnbaum and Maxwell, 1961). A Bayesian analysis was carried out using IPSS data and then replicated using the same probabilities with fresh data from the US–UK project. The results are presented in tables 7.4 and 7.5.

Comparing tables 7.1 and 7.4 it is clear that, based on PSE symptoms only and applied to the IPSS results, the Bayes procedure gives much the same results as Catego. It is therefore worthwhile examining the list of symptoms to discover which have the highest probability of being associated with each diagnosis, and comparing these with the rules in the Catego program. In this way, it will be possible to discover whether the rules laid down in the Catego program have any statistical justification. This exercise will be described in the next section. Comparing tables 7.3 and 7.5, the Bayesian groups are still very highly predictive of clinical diagnosis although not quite so concordant as the Catego classes. This indicates that the sets of probabilities must be very similar in the two series and gives some hope that the diagnostic rules used are also similar. The position is summarised in table 7.6.

Table 7.4. *Diagnostic and Bayesian* classes compared (IPSS series, PSE only)*

IPSS Project diagnosis	Bayesian classes				
	'Schizophrenic and paranoid'	'Manic'	'Depressive'	Total	'Other'
Schizophrenic and paranoid psychoses	690	46	89	825	53
Manic psychoses	8	60	7	75	4
Depressive psychoses and neuroses	10	2	142	154	22
Total	708	108	238	1054	79
Other neuroses and personality disorders	4	–	8	12	41

Excluded: other diagnoses, $N = 16$.
* Using set of probabilities calculated from IPSS data.

Table 7.5. *Diagnostic and Bayesian* classes compared (US–UK series, PSE only)*

IPSS Project diagnosis	Bayesian classes				
	'Schizophrenic and paranoid'	'Manic'	'Depressive'	Total	'Other'
Schizophrenic and paranoid psychoses	187	15	18	220	38
Manic psychoses	15	31	3	49	10
Depressive psychoses and neuroses	34	1	179	214	72
Total	236	47	200	483	120
Other neuroses and personality disorders	13	–	28	41	44

* Using set of probabilities calculated from IPSS data.

Table 7.6. *Prediction of diagnostic groups by Bayesian analysis and by Catego analysis (IPSS and US–UK series, PSE only)*

	IPSS series		US–UK series	
IPSS and US–UK Project diagnosis	Bayesian groups	Catego classes	Bayesian groups	Catego classes
Schizophrenic and paranoid psychoses	78.7	82.0	72.5	74.0
Manic psychoses	76.0	78.5	52.5	66.1
Depressive psychoses and neuroses	80.9	77.3	62.6	80.4
Total	78.9	81.9	65.8	76.3

5. SYMPTOMS DISCRIMINATING SCHIZOPHRENIC AND PARANOID PSYCHOSES

Two sets of probabilities are available: (*a*) the probability that a patient given a particular diagnosis will have a particular symptom, (*b*) the probability that a patient with a particular symptom will be given a particular diagnosis. Thus, using the same three broad diagnostic classes as before, and using symptom no. 3 in list I (worrying) as an example, the two sets of probabilities are as follows:

IPSS Project diagnosis	N	Proportion of those with given diagnosis who have the symptom	Proportion of those with the symptom who are given the diagnosis
Schizophrenic and paranoid psychoses	878	0.58	0.70
Manic psychoses	79	0.57	0.07
Depressive psychoses and neuroses	176	0.74	0.18
Other neuroses	44	0.75	0.05
		(*N* with symptom = 716)	

It is clear that worrying is a very common symptom in IPSS patients: 58% of schizophrenic and paranoid patients worry; so do 57% of manic patients and three-quarters of those with other conditions. The other set of probabilities is therefore of little interest; it merely reflects the proportions of patients in the three diagnostic groups.

In striking contrast is symptom no. 101 in list I (delusions of control):

IPSS Project diagnosis	N	Proportion of those with given diagnosis who have the symptom	Proportion of those with the symptom who are given the diagnosis
Schizophrenic and paranoid psychoses	878	0.25	0.97
Manic psychoses	79	0.05	0.02
Depressive psychoses and neuroses	176	0.02	0.01
Other neuroses	44	–	–
		(N with symptom = 224)	

In this case, the symptom is less frequent but it is present mainly in the schizo-phrenic and paranoid group (in 25% of cases). The second probability shows that the symptom is highly discriminating for one diagnostic group only; 97% of those with the symptom are given a diagnosis of schizophrenic or paranoid psychosis.

The two sets of probabilities had already been calculated for both IPSS and US–UK series, because of the Bayesian analysis. These profiles showed that only four symptoms discriminated at this level (90% or better) in both series. These were (a) delusions of control, (b) thought insertion, broadcast or withdrawal, (c) poverty of content of speech and (d) neologisms. In addition, (e) auditory hallucinations discriminated very well in the IPSS series, and would have done so highly in both series if the different types of hallucination mentioned in section 1 had been rated directly. The probabilities are given, for symptoms in syndrome 1 (NS), in table 7.7.

Symptoms such as neologisms are too rare to be of value in diagnosis, while symptoms such as poverty of content of speech are difficult to illustrate because of language problems. Auditory hallucinations have been discussed earlier; if allowance is made for affectively-based and subculturally-based hallucinations, the probability that the diagnosis will be a schizophrenic or paranoid psychosis becomes 0.96. The cases in which the other two symptoms, 'delusions of control' and 'thought insertion, etc.', were present but a schizophrenic or paranoid psychosis was *not* diagnosed were examined in an attempt to throw light on the discrepancy. Both are first-rank symptoms in Schneider's sense (1971).

DELUSIONS OF CONTROL

Out of 227 patients with this symptom in the entire IPSS series, 96% (218) were diagnosed as suffering from a schizophrenic or paranoid psychosis. The other nine were given diagnoses of mania (296.1 or 296.3, $N = 5$), atypical psychotic depres-

Table 7.7. *Symptoms which are highly discriminating for a diagnosis of schizophrenic or paranoid psychosis (IPPS and US–UK series, PSE only)*

Symptom or syndrome.... {A = IPPS.... B = US–UK.... (N)		Schizophrenic and paranoid psychoses 878 260	Manic psychoses (296.1, 3; 298.1) 79 59	Depressive psychoses (296.0, 2, 8, 9; 298.0) 106 171	Depressive neuroses (300.4) 70 103	Other neuroses (Other 300s) 44 40
96 · Voices to patient*	A 332 B 72	0.93 0.72	0.05 0.04	0.02 0.17	– 0.04	0.01 0.03
97 Voices about patient*	A 173 B 35	0.95 0.89	0.03 0.03	0.02 0.09	– –	– –
98 Commentary by voices*	A 136 B 36	0.95 0.86	0.03 0.06	0.02 0.08	– –	– –
99 Thought broadcast, etc.	A 331 B 73	0.97 0.92	0.02 0.05	0.01 0.03	– –	– –
101 Delusions of control	A 224 B 49	0.97 0.94	0.02 0.02	0.01 0.04	– –	– –

* Symptoms uncorrected for affectively-based or subculturally-based hallucinations.

sion (296.9, $N = 1$; 298.0, $N = 1$), depressive neurosis (300.4, $N = 1$) and hysterical psychosis (298.1, $N = 1$). Brief notes about these patients are given in chapter 11 of IPSS volume 1. In each case, it appeared probable both that the project diagnosis was correct and that the symptom had been incorrectly rated. In one case, for example, the patient thought she was controlled by God. This is a characteristic delusion in manic patients, who do not, however, mean that their will is replaced by that of God, simply that their will seems more powerful than usual, *as though* it were God's. When religious delusions are present as well, they may feel that they are exercising their will according to God's plan, but not that their will is replaced by that of God; on the contrary, they feel their will is magnified. This is a common mistake and the definition in the glossary warns against it. Another interesting discrepancy concerned a Taoist priestess, whose work entailed her giving up her will so that she became possessed by the God. This was a subcultural 'delusion' and would have been rated as such if there had been an appropriate item. The ninth edition has been amended to allow this possibility. The diagnosis of hysterical psychosis was possibly correct. Another kind of reason for the false positive rating was that a patient who was depressed and agitated simply accepted an explanation which she thought was being put forward by the examiner. It was difficult to cross-examine, under the circumstances, and the rating was incorrectly made.

THOUGHT INSERTION, BROADCAST OR WITHDRAWAL

Out of 328 patients with one of these symptoms, 318 (97%) were given a diagnosis of schizophrenic or paranoid psychosis. The other ten were diagnosed as mania (396.1 or 396.3, $N = 6$), depressive psychosis (296.2, $N = 1$; 298.0, $N = 1$), depressive neurosis (300.4, $N = 1$) and hysterical psychosis (298.1, $N = 1$). Four of these patients also had false positive ratings of delusions of control. In these and the other cases it seemed, from the examples given on the PSE schedule, that the symptom had probably not been present and that the ratings were false positives. (Brief notes on each case are given in the appendix.)

CATEGO CLASS S

This class consists of patients with highly discriminating symptoms such as those discussed above, or with auditory hallucinations experienced as speaking *to* the patient in the second person. Out of the 1202 patients in the IPSS series, 563 (47%) were placed into class S. If allowance is made for the rating of false positive symptoms discussed above, and for the mistaking of affectively-based and sub-culturally-based hallucinations, it appears possible that this class, when derived from correct ratings, constitutes a core group within the diagnostic category of schizophrenia, and that whatever pathology is ultimately discovered to be associated with it must account in a satisfactory way for the form of these very highly discriminating symptoms.

This does not mean, of course, that the highly discriminating symptoms are the only ones present in the clinical picture of patients with schizophrenic and paranoid illnesses. On the contrary, if syndrome 1 (NS) is omitted, nearly all of these patients are still placed into classes S or P by the Catego program, because of the presence of other characteristic syndromes. Even if both syndrome 1 (NS) and syndrome 13 (AH) are omitted, the Catego class of patients diagnosed as schizophrenic or paranoid usually remains concordant (P+, P?, O+, O?). Thus although these symptoms are highly specific, the diagnosis does not depend *only* upon them.

6. SYMPTOMS DISCRIMINATING AFFECTIVE DIAGNOSES

No symptom within list I discriminates any of the affective diagnoses with the power of those mentioned in section 5. The most useful predictor of a diagnosis of manic psychosis (296.1, 296.3, 298.1 reactive excitement) is 12 (HM), with its constituent symptoms; subjective euphoria, ideomotor pressure, elation at the time of interview and flight of ideas. Other useful syndromes are 16 (GR) and 20 (OV). However, all these syndromes are quite frequently rated as present in schizophrenic patients. Symptom no. 44 (subjective euphoria), which is rated present in 228 IPSS cases altogether, occurs in 154 schizophrenic and paranoid patients (67.5%), so that it is hardly a useful predictor of mania in this series. In the US–UK series, which contains relatively fewer schizophrenic patients, out of 78 patients with the symptom only 23 are schizophrenic, but only 30 are diagnosed as manic. If, on the other hand, patients with a diagnosis of schizophrenia are omitted from consideration, a symptom such as 44, subjective euphoria becomes more highly discriminating of a diagnosis of mania (86.5% in the IPSS series, for example).

Table 7.8 combines data from the IPSS and US–UK series in order to achieve reasonable numbers on which to base probabilities. Patients with a diagnosis of schizophrenic or paranoid psychosis are omitted from consideration in the calculation of probabilities and, in this way, the probability of predicting a diagnosis of manic psychosis is seen to be quite high using certain symptoms and syndromes.

In the same way, the most discriminating symptoms for a diagnosis of depressive psychosis can only be detected after the schizophrenic and paranoid conditions have been excluded. The symptoms constituting syndromes 5 (DD), 6 (SD) and 24 (ED) have the highest probabilities. Thus syndrome 6 (SD) was rated as present in 1494 patients in the IPSS and US–UK series but, of these, 868 (58%) were given schizophrenic or paranoid diagnoses. Considering only the 626 others, 42% were given a diagnosis of psychotic depression, 27% of neurotic depression, 18% of other neurosis and 13% of mania. The delusional syndrome, 5 (DD), is naturally more predictive of psychotic depression (66 out of 84 patients with the syndrome, or 79%) than of the other affective conditions.

The most important point to emphasise here is that a major principle on which clinicians make a diagnosis is hierarchical. First-rank schizophrenic symptoms are

Table 7.8. *Symptoms which discriminate a diagnosis of manic psychosis when schizophrenic and paranoid psychoses are excluded (IPSS and US–UK series, PSE only)*

Symptom or syndrome* (A = IPSS... / B = US–UK...)	(N)	Schizophrenic and paranoid psychoses 878 / 260	Manic psychoses 79 / 59	Depressive psychoses 106 / 171	Depressive neuroses 70 / 103	Other neuroses 44 / 40	N with affective conditions 299 / 273
44 Subjective euphoria	A 228 / B 78	154 / 23	0.76	0.10	0.09	0.05	124
45 Ideomotor pressure	A 159 / B 89	94 / 26	0.82	0.11	0.03	0.03	122
46 Grandiose ideas	A 177 / B 50	113 / 21	0.92	0.07	–	0.01	86
84 Elation	A 135 / B 53	75 / 22	0.94	0.06	0.01	–	93
137 Flight of ideas	A 91 / B 35	63 / 13	0.94	0.04	0.02	–	48
Syndrome 12 (HM)	A 355 / B 151	259 / 54	0.68	0.15	0.08	0.09	185
Syndrome 16 (GR)	A 264 / B 57	217 / 41	0.92	0.06	–	0.02	63
Syndrome 20 (OV)	A 107 / B 40	87 / 21	0.87	0.08	–	0.05	39

* Only syndromes with a (+) or (++) degree of certainty are included.

105

given higher weight than, say, subjective euphoria or depression and these, in turn, are given greater weight than worrying. If there are no first-rank symptoms, however, then symptoms lower in the hierarchy are given greater weight in arriving at the diagnosis, and so on down the list of priorities. This is the main principle behind the Catego system also. It would be instructive to attempt a refinement and simplification of the Catego rule system, using this hierarchical principle and a series of Bayesian analyses at each level. For the moment, however, the value of the Catego system is that the rules have been worked out clinically, not statistically.

7. THE ADDITION OF DATA FROM THE CLINICAL HISTORY

The Catego program provides, in stage 10, for the addition of clinical information (in the form of ratings of syndromes made from data in case-notes or from informants) to that contained in the PSE. The descriptive class derived on the basis of the historical information can be combined with that derived from the PSE data to give a modified descriptive grouping which should presumably be somewhat more valid than the class based on PSE data alone.

In order to test the reliability of this procedure, an exercise was undertaken using the narrative histories written about IPSS patients. These varied very widely in length and content; some centres supplying detailed accounts, others submitting brief but precise notes and yet others containing only minimal information. One rater (J. W.) had already looked at the records of all discrepant and uncertain cases and a proportion of concordant ones, omitting only those placed into class S on PSE data alone, since the categorisation in these cases could not be changed by the addition of material from the clinical history. (The terms 'discrepant', 'uncertain' and 'concordant' describe the degree of agreement between Catego class and Centre diagnosis and will be considered in more detail in section 8.) A second rater (Dr Ctirad Skoda, from Prague) was then asked to make independent ratings on the syndrome check list of a random one-in-ten sample of the IPSS series (all those with a case-number ending in 0) and a further one-in-ten sample selected so as to contain equal numbers of concordant, uncertain and discrepant cases. The results using the two groups were closely similar and they have therefore been combined, giving a total of 239 cases, i.e. a 20% sample of 1202, with one case omitted because the notes had been mislaid. Of these, 134 histories were rated by both examiners. The syndrome ratings were used to derive descriptive Catego classes and table 7.9 contains a comparison of the 134 cases rated by both C.S. and J.W.

There is a considerable degree of agreement between the two raters. In terms of the simple three-way classification used earlier (S, O, P/M/D, R, N), 105 cases are agreed out of 134 (78.4%). If only the five Centres with fairly detailed narrative histories are considered, this proportion becomes 86.1%. In view of the unstandardised and often scanty information available, this degree of reliability was very encouraging.

Table 7.9. *Descriptive Catego classes derived from syndrome ratings of two examiners (IPSS series, SCL data; rated by C.S. and J.W.)*

Catego class (SCL rated by J.W.)	Catego class (SCL rated by C.S.)								
	S	P	O	M	D	R	N	A, B, H, X	Total
S	13	1	1	–	–	–	–	–	15
P	8	19	4	3	1	1	5	2	43
O	1	–	5	–	1	–	–	1	8
M	–	3	2	11	–	–	1	–	17
D	–	1	–	1	6	1	–	–	9
R	–	–	–	2	1	5	2	2	12
N	1	1	1	–	2	7	8	3	23
A, B, H, X	1	–	1	–	–	–	–	5	7
Total	24	25	14	17	11	14	16	13	134

Table 7.10 presents a comparison between the distributions when Skoda's SCL ratings have been added. The main change occurs in the uncertain classes; out of 37 cases, 23 become more certainly classified and only 14 remain queries. In addition, many of the patients classified as 'neurotic' on PSE data alone, are given a definite psychotic classification when historical data are added. Those who were fairly definitely classified as psychotic, however, tend to change classification very little. In fact, the overall changes introduced by adding material from the history are not great, a conclusion similar to that reached by Simon *et al.* (1971).

The results of this exercise appeared to indicate that it would be reasonable to use the SCL ratings of the IPSS narrative case-histories in order to supplement the PSE data available and provide a descriptive classification based upon more complete data. A more important conclusion may also be drawn; that if historical data were deliberately collected in a standard fashion, the resulting Catego classification would be correspondingly more useful. In fact, as Skoda (personal communication) points out, the PH data could become the main input for classification, with the PSE data serving by way of correction.

The remaining tables in this chapter are therefore based upon the classification using PSE and historical data (rated by J.W.) combined.

8. DIAGNOSTIC AND CATEGO CLASSES COMPARED

It has already been demonstrated (see tables 7.1, 7.2 and 7.3) that there is a substantial relationship between diagnostic class and Catego class based on PSE data alone. Table 7.11 shows that there is an even stronger relationship when historical data are added.

Table 7.10. *Comparison of Catego classification using PSE data alone, with classification after SCL data have been added (20% sample of IPSS series; Skoda's ratings of SCL)*

Catego class (PSE only)	Catego class (PSE+PH)								
	S	P+	O+	M+	D+	P?, O?, M?, D?	R, N	A, B, H, X	Total
S	94	–	–	–	–	1	–	–	95
P+	3	14	–	–	–	–	–	–	17
O+	1	–	4	–	–	–	–	–	5
M+	2	–	–	18	–	–	–	–	20
D+	2	–	–	–	13	–	–	–	15
D+	7	5	3	6	2	14	–	–	37
P?, O?, M?, D?	3	1	2	3	2	2	23	–	36
R, N	2	1	2	1	–	1	1	6	14
A, B, H, X									
Total	114	21	11	28	17	18	24	6	239

Table 7.11. *Diagnostic and Catego classes compared (IPSS series, PSE+PH)*

IPSS Project diagnosis	Catego class (PSE+PH)				A, B, H, X
	S, O, P	M	D, R, N	Total	
Schizophrenic and paranoid psychoses	786	44	46	876	2
Manic psychoses	10	66	3	79	–
Depressive psychoses and neuroses	35	13	128	176	–
Total	831	123	177	1131	2
Other neuroses and personality disorders	8	4	32	44	–

Excluded: Personality disorders ($N = 9$) and other diagnoses ($N = 16$).

In terms of a crude three-way classification, the degree of concordance is clearly very high (87%, coefficient of contingency $C = 0.68$). The χ^2 test, of course, rejects the null hypothesis of no association in the table ($\chi^2 = 960.3$, d.f. = 4, $P < 0.001$) but this information is of limited value since it is obvious by inspection.

Maxwell's test for differences between the lateral totals (Maxwell, 1970) shows that the proportions of cases in the three groups produced by the Catego and diagnostic systems are, in fact, significantly different ($\chi^2 = 25.0$, d.f. = 2, $P < 0.001$).

Furthermore, Maxwell gives a test for the hypothesis that the population values of the corresponding off-diagonal terms are equal. This also is rejected ($\chi^2 = 25.5$, d.f. = 3, $P < 0.001$) which means that significantly more cases are diagnosed as schizophrenic by Centre psychiatrists but not placed into class S, than are identified as class S by the Catego program but diagnosed as manic or depressive. The 'bias' therefore is towards schizophrenia diagnosed by Centre psychiatrists (or towards affective conditions identified by the Catego program). The reasons for a possible over-diagnosing of schizophrenia will be discussed in section 10 below.

However, the immediate impression from table 7.11 is of a very substantial agreement between the two systems.

9. ASSESSMENT OF USEFULNESS: THE 'BASE RATE'

As Meehl and Rosen (1955) have pointed out, the question of statistical significance should be separated from that of usefulness. 'Since diagnostic and prognostic statements can often be made with a high degree of accuracy purely on the basis of actuarial or experience tables (referred to hereinafter as *base rates*), a psychometric device, to be efficient, must make possible a greater number of correct decisions than could be made in terms of the base rates alone.' They make the same point more succinctly as follows, 'Results are frequently reported only in terms of significance tests for differences between groups rather than in terms of the number of correct decisions for individuals within the groups.'

Meehl and Rosen point out that it is perfectly possible, by the use of a diagnostic test which is significantly associated with the criterion in statistical terms, actually to *decrease* one's ability to predict. Consider, for example, the following table:

	Test result	
Diagnosis	Condition A	Condition B
Condition A	65	15
Condition B	10	10

These results show a significant association between a diagnosis of condition A or B and the results of a diagnostic test. However, since 80 of the 100 patients are diagnosed as having condition A, an excellent prediction can be made by assuming that *all* the patients have condition A. In this way, 80 patients will be correctly identified at the cost of 20 false positives. The use of the test actually decreases predictability, since only 75 of the patients are concordantly classified by using it, instead of 80 without it. Such a result is only acceptable if it is of great importance to identify at least some of the patients with condition B, but less urgent to diagnose those with condition A. If condition B were a brain tumour and condition A absence of a brain tumour, it would be better to use the test as a screening device, since it picks out 10 of the 20 patients with condition B while the base rate picks out none. These results are a simple consequence of Bayes' rule. Meehl and Rosen conclude that the best policy is to 'follow the base rates when they are better than the test', unless there is some specifiable reason to the contrary.

So far as the results in this chapter are concerned, there is no particular reason to suppose that it is more important to identify one diagnostic group rather than another and the arguments of Meehl and Rosen are apposite. (As a matter of fact Bayes' rule always applies, and what changes is the decision problem to which it is applied.)

It is worth emphasising, however, that terms such as 'hit rate', 'false positive', etc., imply values which have not been demonstrated to be correct. The Catego classification has as great a chance of being 'right' (in the sense of being valid according to some external criterion such as predicting aetiology, response to treatment, or outcome) as the diagnostic system with which it is compared. The terms 'concordance' and 'discrepancy' will therefore be used throughout, to designate agreement and disagreement.

Meehl and Rosen point out that it is easiest to improve on a base rate decision policy when base rates are close to a fifty–fifty split. Table 7.11 shows that, out of

1131 patients, 876 (77.5%) are diagnosed as having schizophrenic or paranoid psychoses. Thus, if it were assumed that every patient in the series suffered from a schizophrenic or a paranoid psychosis, only 22.5% would be classified discrepantly with Centre diagnosis. The Catego classification does, however, improve upon this by about 9.2%:

Diagnostic class	N	Base rate concordance N	Base rate concordance %	Catego concordance N	Catego concordance %
Schizophrenic and paranoid psychoses	876	876	100.0	786	89.7
Manic psychoses	79	0	–	66	83.5
Depressive psychoses and neuroses	176	0	–	128	72.7
Overall	1131	876	77.5	980	86.7 (3-way)
				996	88.1 (2-way)

In addition, the Catego classification distinguishes usefully between manic and depressive conditions, which the overall base rate cannot do at all.

However, Meehl and Rosen make one further important point: 'If a psychometric test is applied solely to the criterion groups from which it was developed, its reported validity and efficiency is likely to be spuriously high, especially if the criterion groups are small.' In the present case, the criterion groups are of reasonable size, but the general stricture is cogent. However, the US–UK series presents an opportunity to compare diagnostic and Catego classes in a material which was not used for the development of the Catego program. Only the UK data have been used in table 7.12 because the brief narrative histories were readily available for this group and syndrome ratings could be made. This table is directly comparable with table 7.3. The concordances are as follows:

Diagnostic class	N	Base rate concordance N	Base rate concordance %	Catego concordance N	Catego concordance %
Schizophrenic and paranoid psychoses	118	0	–	111	94.1
Manic psychoses	26 ⎫	190	100.0	19	73.1
Depressive psychoses and neuroses	164 ⎭			139	84.8
Overall	308	190	61.7	269	87.3 (3-way)
				283	91.9 (2-way)

Table 7.12. *Diagnostic and Catego classes compared (UK series, PSE+PH)*

| UK series Project diagnosis | Catego class (PSE+PH) | | | | A, B, H, X |
	S, O, P	M	D, R, N	Total	
Schizophrenic and paranoid psychoses	111	1	6	118	2
Manic psychoses	7	19	–	26	–
Depressive psychoses and neuroses	11	14	139	164	–
Total	129	34	145	308	2
Other neuroses and personality disorders	1	5	29	–	6

As Meehl and Rosen stated, it is much easier to beat the base rate when it is close to symmetry, but the essential finding is that the concordance between the Catego classification and the US–UK Project diagnostic groups is quite as high as it is with the IPSS Project diagnoses.

10. CATEGO CLASSES COMPARED WITH FOUR-FIGURE ICD RUBRICS

Table 7.13 presents a comparison of the individual four-figure ICD diagnoses used in the IPSS series with Catego classes based on information from the PSE and psychiatric history combined.

It is clear that, from a purely symptomatological point of view, many of the specific diagnoses do not seem to have a characteristic clinical picture. The diagnosis may be made on criteria such as supposed aetiology (e.g. reactive excitement or reactive confusion) or possibly on previous personality (e.g. simple or latent schizophrenia). Volume 1 of the IPSS report gives profiles of four digit ICD categories.

The diagnoses are grouped together in table 7.14 according to their Catego class composition. There is a group of four subcategories of schizophrenia (295.3, 295.4, 295.1, and 295.7) which appear difficult to separate from each other using this technique and which are mainly characterised by class S symptoms. Another group consists of rarely used diagnoses which are more difficult to standardise because they are rag bag categories (295.8, 295.9, 298.9, 299 etc.). There is a small paranoid group (297.0, 297.9) which is strongly related to class P. The other four subcategories of schizophrenia (295.0, 295.2, 295.5, 295.6) appear to be characterised by class S symptoms in a considerable proportion of cases but there is a discrete group with class O symptoms, mainly accounted for by catatonic schizophrenia, 295.2.

Table 7.13. *Specific ICD rubrics compared with Catego classification (IPSS series: PSE+PH)*

ICD Rubric		Catego classes (PSE+PH)											Total
		S	P+	P?	O+	O?	M+	M?	D+	D?	R	N	
Schizophrenic psychoses													
295.0	Simple schizophrenia	12	1	4	9	–	–	1	–	–	1	3	31
295.1	Hebeph. schizophrenia	62	8	5	3	–	5	2	–	–	–	1	86
295.2	Catat. schizophrenia	26	2	3	19	–	2	1	–	–	–	1	54
295.3	Paranoid schizophrenia	260	39	12	4	–	4	2	–	–	–	–	321
295.4	Acute schizophrenia	57	1	2	4	1	4	3	2	–	–	–	74
295.5	Latent schizophrenia	8	–	–	–	1	1	1	–	–	1	–	12
	Sluggish schizophrenia	–	–	–	1	–	4	–	1	–	–	6	12
295.6	Residual schizophrenia	7	1	2	–	–	–	–	–	–	2	3	15
295.7	Schiz.-aff. psychosis	71	11	5	1	1	7	–	4	1	2	4	107
295.8	Other schizophrenias	6	–	2	2	–	1	–	–	–	–	–	11
295.9	Schiz. NOS	27	6	9	1	–	–	2	2	–	–	–	47
–	Shift-like schiz.	17	3	2	1	–	1	1	2	–	2	4	33
–	Periodic schizophrenia	2	–	–	–	–	2	–	1	1	–	–	6
													809
Paranoid psychoses													
297.0	Paranoia	–	1	1	–	–	–	–	–	–	–	–	2
297.9	Other para. psychosis	6	7	1	–	–	–	–	–	–	–	–	14
298.2	Reac. confusion	1	2	1	–	–	–	–	–	–	–	1	4
298.3	Ps. para. reaction	6	1	1	–	–	–	–	–	–	–	–	8
298.9	Reac. Ps. NOS	5	3	2	–	1	–	–	1	–	–	–	12
299	Psychosis NOS	–	1	–	–	–	–	–	–	–	–	–	1
–	Psychogen. par. psychosis	8	3	1	–	–	–	–	1	–	–	–	13
–	Acute par. psychosis	8	2	3	–	–	–	–	1	–	–	–	13
													67

Table 7.13 (continued)

ICD rubric		Catego classes (PSE+PH)											Total
		S	P+	P?	O+	O?	M+	M?	D+	D?	R	N	
Manic psychoses													
296.1	Mania	6	1	–	–	–	56	1	1	–	–	1	66
296.3	Circular psychoses	3	–	–	–	–	8	–	1	–	–	–	12
298.1	Reac. excitement	–	–	–	–	–	1	–	–	–	–	–	1 79
Depressive psychoses and neuroses													
296.0	Invol. melancholia	1	1	1	1	–	1	–	1	–	–	–	5
296.2	Ps. depression	3	4	4	1	–	7	2	31	–	13	8	73
296.8	Other aff. psychoses	–	–	–	–	–	1	–	1	–	–	–	1
296.9	Aff. Ps. NOS	2	3	–	–	–	1	–	–	–	–	–	6
298.0	Reac. depression	3	–	4	–	–	–	–	4	1	3	6	21
300.4	Neur. depression	2	–	6	–	–	2	–	7	–	17	36	70 176
	Total	609	100	71	47	4	107	16	58	3	40	76	1131

*Omitted cases**

300.1–3, 5–9	Other neuroses	44
301.1–9	Pers. disorders	9
298.1	Hysterical ps.	6
294.4	Puerperal ps.	8
–	?Epilepsy	2
		69

* Two patients in other Catego classes are also omitted; one diagnosed 295.5 (Centre 6), the other 298.9 (Centre 3).

Table 7.14. *Groups of ICD diagnoses compared with Catego classification IPSS (PSE + PH)*

	ICD rubrics	S	P	O	M	D, R, N	Total %	(N)
				Catego classes (%)				
1	295.3 Paranoid S.	81	16	1	2	–	100	(321)
	295.4 Acute S.	77	4	5	10	4	100	(74)
	295.1 Hebephrenic S.	72	15	4	8	1	100	(86)
	295.7 Schizo-affective	66	15	2	7	10	100	(107)
2	295.8, 9; Shift-like S, Periodic S.	54	23	5	7	11	100	(97)
	298.2, 3, 9; 299; PPP; APP.	55	37	2	–	6	100	(51)
3	297.0; 297.9	38	63	–	–	–	101	(16)
4	295.0, 2, 5, (5), 6	43	10	25	8	14	100	(124)
5	296.1, 3; 298.1	11	1	–	84	4	100	(79)
6	296.2	4	11	1	12	71	99	(73)
	300.4	3	9	–	3	86	101	(70)
7	296.0, 8, 9; 298.0	18	27	–	6	48	99	(33)
	Total (N)	609	171	51	123	177		1131

The manic psychoses (296.1, 296.3 and 298.1, reactive excitement) are equivalent to class M. The depressive psychoses and neuroses are notoriously difficult to classify and there is considerable overlap. In particular, there is no possibility, in the ICD, of distinguishing between patients in Catego classes R and N (retarded and neurotic depression). The rubric 296.2, psychotic depression, may include both 'psychotic' conditions, in the sense of patients with delusions or stupor, and 'endogenous' conditions, in the sense of retardation, guilt, etc. The rubrics 296.0, involutional melancholia and 298.0, reactive depressive psychosis, may include patients with marked degrees of anxiety and thus overlap to some extent with neurotic depression. Thus class D may be regarded as equivalent to a part of 296.2, and class N to 300.4, but class R might be allocated either way according to the varying diagnostic rules of different clinicians. It has no 'psychotic' content but it is characterised by retardation. Allowing for this difficulty in the ICD, there is a fair degree of association with the Catego classification. Table 7.15 shows the combined data from the IPSS and UK series, utilising data from the PSE and psychiatric history. Considering only the diagnoses 296.2 and 300.4, 53 out of 60 class D patients (88.3%) are given the former rubric, and 82 out of 114 class N patients (71.9%) are given the latter. Class R patients are distributed almost equally between the diagnoses.

Table 7.15. *Subclassification of the affective disorders (IPSS and UK series, PSE+PH)*

ICD diagnosis	Catego class (PSE+PH)				
	M	D	R	N	Total
296.1, 296.3, 298.1	85	2	–	1	88
296.2	15	53	34	32	134
300.4	8	7	28	82	125
296.0, 8, 9; 298.0	4	10	10	12	36
Total	112	72	72	127	383

The only data available on other Catego classes are concerned with class A. In Binitie's material 49 patients were given a diagnosis of 300.0, anxiety state, and 39 of these (79.6%) were placed in class A by the Catego program. There were no 'false positives' in this class. The differentiation was from mania (10 cases) and depression (88 cases).

11. LESSONS TO BE LEARNED FROM DISCREPANT AND UNCERTAIN CLASSIFICATIONS

In all IPSS cases where the Catego class based on PSE combined with PH data remained uncertain (94 out of 1131, 8%) or discrepant (105 out of 1131, or 9%) with the project diagnosis, an examination was made of all the material available, including the narrative histories and the examples of ratings written on the PSE schedules. The reasons for discrepancies could be divided into five groups.

The first of these contains cases such as those discussed at the beginning of this chapter, where the discrepancy is due to the schedule items not reflecting adequately the diversity of the symptoms to be rated. The most obvious example in the IPSS series was auditory hallucinations which was dealt with by amending the interview schedule. The ninth edition should be able to cope with these particular symptoms.

The second major group has been considered in section 5; it contains patients who were rated as showing a symptom but who very probably did not, in fact, have it. The only way to overcome such problems is to ensure that raters all know the nature of the symptoms they are looking for. The glossary of definitions should help this process of training.

A third group contained patients who appeared to be discrepantly classified because of coding errors. There were very few of these but they were striking. For example, the clinical formulation in one case was, 'A depressive state with delusional ideas of self-accusation, motor and speech retardation, derealisation symptoms, suicidal thoughts and attempts, sleeping and appetite disturbances'. The Catego class was D+ which appears to be concordant. The actual diagnosis recorded, however, was schizophrenia.

The fourth group contained cases that were quite simply difficult to diagnose. Most obvious, perhaps, were cases with a mixture of symptoms with different diagnostic implications; paranoid and depressive, for example, or excited and elated. Many of the cases in this group would always lead to a good deal of disagreement between psychiatrists, and it is unlikely that any one set of rules would obtain universal assent.

In the final group of discrepant cases the clinician had clearly taken into account data which were not included in the Catego input. The main item was change in personality, particularly towards indifference and isolation, which appeared sometimes to be used to indicate a diagnosis of schizophrenia irrespective of other symptomatology. The problem of reducing the number of such discrepancies lies entirely in the standardisation of what constitutes a personality change of diagnostic significance. Certain schools of thought lay great emphasis on this and it is their responsibility to define the changes involved and demonstrate that they can be rated reliably. Certain diagnoses are particularly affected, e.g. latent, borderline, pseudo-neurotic and simple schizophrenia.

Thus three of these five groups can be reduced in size to some extent, by using better schedules, giving better training and by careful examination to eliminate coding errors. Considerable technical work will be necessary before the other two kinds of problem are solved. However, the number of discrepancies overall is not very large (9%).

An examination of cases with an uncertain classification (P?, O?, M?, D?) even when information from the psychiatric history has been added also yields useful lessons about how to improve the quality of a computer-simulated diagnostic process. In the first place, however, it should be pointed out that the Catego classification is often broadly concordant even though uncertain. Of the 71 patients in class P?, for example, 56 were given a clinical diagnosis of schizophrenic or paranoid psychosis, leaving only 15 discrepant cases. The most important reason for uncertainty may well be lack of information. Many of the narrative histories were very brief or lacking in specific clinical content. The development of the syndrome check list will do much to improve this situation. However, the next commonest reason for an uncertain classification appeared to be a realistic one, that the cases were indeed difficult to diagnose and even with excellent information available it would be difficult to come to a certain conclusion. The main category to note here is the group of patients with 'monosymptomatic' delusions. One patient thought he was accused of being homosexual, another thought he was giving off an unpleasant smell, another thought her facial appearance was changing. Apart from these fragmentary delusions there were no psychotic symptoms. Psychiatrists disagree as to how such cases should be classified. Another group of cases had only 'subcultural' delusions, e.g. a Nigerian man might say that he was being attacked by witchcraft but have no other 'delusional' symptoms. The change in the ninth edition of the PSE which makes it possible to separate such symptoms should deal with such problems. In a few cases the psychotic symptom rated as present was probably rated in error; usually this was when a neurotic symptom presented in a rather unusual way and was rated as a partial delusion.

Thus an examination of the uncertainly classified cases brings up the same sort of problems as the study of discrepancies and gives rise to the same sorts of suggestion as to how the problems can be solved.

12. CHARACTERISTICS OF CATEGO CLASSES

Syndrome profiles of the main Catego classes are presented as figures 7.1–7.7.* Uncertain classes are combined with the relevant more certain class, e.g. P? and P+ are combined as class P. In each case, the profiles for IPSS and US–UK data are compared and it is clear that there is a very close resemblance. The US–UK clinicians tend to rate relatively fewer psychotic syndromes and relatively more neurotic syndromes as present but the shapes of the profiles are nevertheless remarkably concordant. This is not only true of those syndromes which define the particular class. For example, class S is defined only in terms of syndromes 1 (NS) and 13 (AH), but the shape of the 20-syndrome profile is closely similar in the two quite independently rated series.

Product-moment correlation coefficients were calculated, using a modified form of the logit transformation to take account of zero frequencies. In each case the correlation coefficient for 35 syndromes was 0.83 or better. The actual values are shown on the appropriate figures.

No data are at present available to illustrate the clinical picture of classes H (hysterical conditions) and B (obsessional neuroses). The 50-class grouping does of course allow a much finer differentiation and each of the 50 has its own symdrome profile.

The clinical characteristics of the broad Catego classes will now be summarised using the data presented in this chapter.

CLASS S+. SCHIZOPHRENIC PSYCHOSES

This class contains the central schizophrenic conditions. The characteristic symptoms are:
  (i) thought intrusion, broadcast or withdrawal,
  (ii) delusions of control,
  (iii) voices discussing patient in third person or commenting on thoughts or actions,

* See appendix for syndromes.

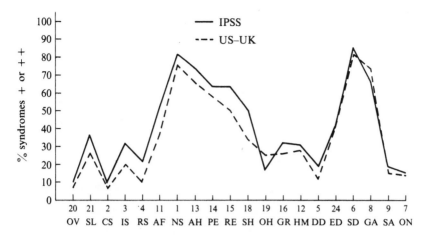

Figure 7.1. Syndrome profiles, class S ($r = 0.85$).

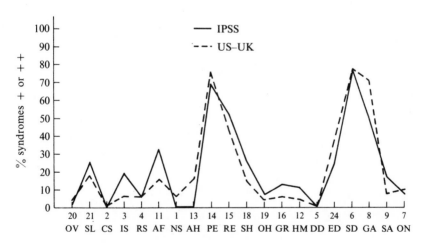

Figure 7.2. Syndrome profiles, class P ($r = 0.95$).

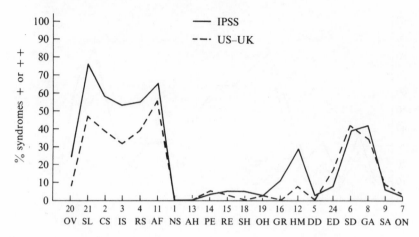

Figure 7.3. Syndrome profiles, class O ($r = 0.85$).

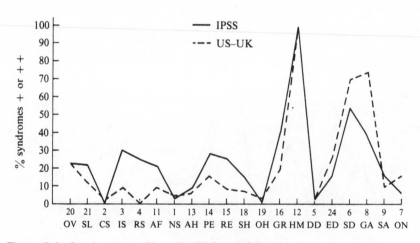

Figure 7.4. Syndrome profiles, class M ($r = 0.83$).

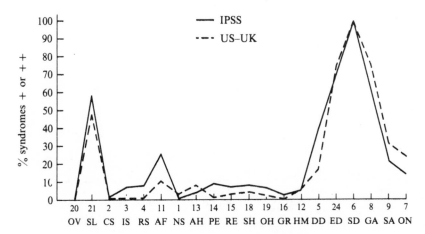

Figure 7.5. Syndrome profiles, classes D+R ($r = 0.93$).

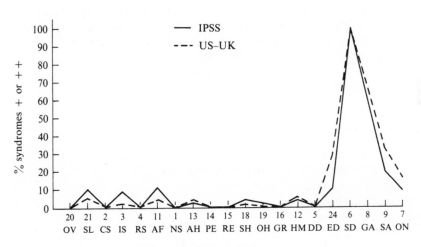

Figure 7.6. Syndrome profiles, class N ($r = 0.96$).

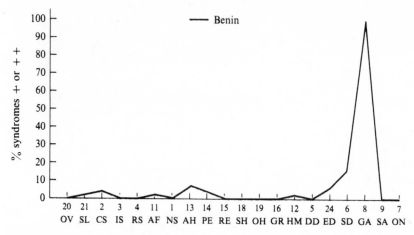

Figure 7.7. Syndrome profile, class A.

(iv) other auditory hallucinations (not affectively based),

(v) other delusions.

If any of the first three symptoms is present the patient is automatically allo-' cated to class S+; similarly if *both* symptoms (iv) and (v) are present. Schizo-affective subclasses can be distinguished. Over half the patients in the IPSS series were placed into this class. A high proportion of these patients were given a diagnosis of paranoid (81%), acute (77%), hebephrenic (72%) or schizo-affective (66%) schizophrenia. Clearly this is a conservative estimate, since various other kinds of primary phenomena are not included and information from the clinical history usually understates the frequency of first rank symptoms in previous episodes.

CLASS M+. MANIC AND MIXED AFFECTIVE PSYCHOSES

The chief symptoms are:

(i)   subjective euphoria, or elation on examination,

(ii)   ideomotor pressure,

(iii) grandiose ideas,

(iv)   grandiose delusions,

(v)   flight of ideas,

(vi)   overactivity.

The first symptom must be present together with at least one other, in the absence of symptoms from class S+. A hypomanic subclass can be distinguished. Mixed affective conditions are included. Of patients given a diagnosis of mania in the IPSS series (296.1, 296.3 or 298.1), 82% are in class M+.

CLASS D+. DEPRESSIVE PSYCHOSES

The chief symptoms are:
  (i) depressed mood,
  (ii) depressive delusions or hallucinations.

Both symptoms must be present, in the absence of symptoms of class S+ or M+. The commonest diagnosis given to patients in this class is 296.2.

CLASS P+. PARANOID PSYCHOSES

The chief symptoms are:
  (i) delusions (other than first-rank),
  (ii) hallucinations (other than auditory).

This class contains patients with delusions and hallucinations other than those characteristic of classes S+, M+ or D+. Diagnoses associated particularly with class P+ are 297.0 and 297.9 (paranoid psychoses).

CLASS O+. OTHER PSYCHOSES

The chief symptoms are:
  (i) catatonic symptoms
  (ii) behaviour indicates hallucinations.

Patients are allocated to this class only if there are no other psychotic symptoms. This class is mainly represented in two diagnostic subgroups, simple schizophrenia (295.0) and catatonic schizophrenia (295.2). Only 47 out of 1131 patients in the IPSS series were allocated to this class.

UNCERTAIN PSYCHOTIC CLASSES (S?, P?, M?, D?)

Each of the main psychotic classes has a less certain counterpart.

  S? Voices experienced as speaking directly to the patient, but not characteristic of depression or mania, constitute the only psychotic symptom present.

  M? The symptoms are similar to those of class M+ but there is minimal euphoria or elation.

  D? This class is rarely used. It contains, for example, patients with depressed mood and olfactory hallucinations only.

  P? This is the only common uncertain psychotic class. It contains cases with delusions of persecution or reference in the absence of more diagnostic symptoms and patients with only 'partial' delusions.

CLASS R. RETARDED DEPRESSION

The chief symptoms are:
  (i)   depressed mood,
  (ii) retardation,
  (iii) guilt, self-depreciation, etc.
  (iv) agitation.

The first of these symptoms must be present, together with one of the others, in the absence of depressive delusions or other psychotic symptoms. In the combined IPSS and UK series, class R cases were distributed approximately equally between the diagnoses 296.2 and 300.4.

CLASS N. NEUROTIC DEPRESSIONS

The chief symptoms are:
  (i) depressed mood,
  (ii) anxiety.

The first symptom must be present, in the absence of psychotic symptoms or symptoms characteristic of class R. Most patients are diagnosed as 300.4.

CLASS A. ANXIETY STATES

The chief symptoms are:
  (i)   subjective or observed anxiety,
  (ii) situational anxiety (e.g. fear of crowds),
  (iii) specific anxiety (e.g. fear of birds).

Patients are allocated to this class only if depressive symptoms are not predominant and no psychotic symptoms are present. In one series with a fairly large number of patients diagnosed as 300.0 (anxiety state), the Catego program placed nearly all into class A, differentiating them from depressive and manic conditions.

OTHER CLASSES

No series is available with large enough numbers of patients with obsessional conditions or hysteria to test whether the Catego program differentiates these conditions. There is a residual class X, into which patients who have only non-specific symptoms such as worrying are placed. Finally, class O? is used so rarely when historical information is available that it can be ignored.

13. THE 50-CLASS GROUPING

The major classes described in section 12 can be broken down into 50 subclasses. The constituent elements (taken from table 6.4) are shown in table 7.15, together with their frequencies in the IPSS series. Clearly these could be reconstituted in various ways; for example, all the subclasses which combine a schizophrenic or paranoid component with a manic or psychotic depressive component could be combined to give a large schizo-affective class (NSMN/DSMN, NSPD/DSPD, DPMN, DPPD, CSMN, CSPD, RSMN, RSPD, MNCS, MNRS, PDRS). The schizo-manic subclasses could be separated from the schizo-depressive. The syndrome profiles of these various classes can be predicted quite closely from combining the appropriate profiles shown in figures 7.1–7.5.

Smaller subclasses such as NS+, DS+, CS+, RS+, DP+ and DP? may have specific interest in their own right. Subclasses DP+ and DP? might very well be subdivided further, although the numbers involved are relatively small. The same is true of subclasses such as AN+ and PN+.

Table 7.15. *Fifty Catego subclasses and their frequencies IPSS (PSE+PH)*, $N = 1202$

Major class	Subclasses	N		%
S+	1 NS+	431		
	2 NS?	17		
	3 DS+	100	593	49.4
	22 NSMN/DSMN	26		
	29 NSPD	19		
S?	4 DS?	19		1.6
P+	5 DP+	81		
	23 DPMN	14	102	8.5
	30 DPPD	7		
P?	6 DP?	66	74	6.2
	31 DP?/AP?	8		
O+	7 CS+	27		
	8 RS+	8		
	26 CSMN	8	49	4.1
	28 RSMN	3		
	33 RSPD	–		
	34 CSPD	3		
O?	9 RS?	–		
	10 SS	2		
	17 UP+	2	5	0.4
	18 UP?	1		
	35 XP	–		

Table 7.15 (*continued*)

Major class	Subclasses	N	%
M+	13 MN+	72	
	21 MAP+	18	
	15 HM+	22 } 112	9.3
	25 MNCS	–	
	27 MNRS	–	
M?	14 MN?	16	1.3
D+	11 PD+	60 } 60	5.0
	19 AP+	–	
D?	12 PD?	1	
	20 AP?	2 } 3	0.3
	32 PDRS	–	
R+	42 RD+	42	3.5
N+	38 ND+	24 } 97	8.1
	40 SD+	73	
N?	39 ND?	–	
	41 SD?	3 } 10	0.8
	43 RD?	7	
A+	44 AN+	4 } 6	0.5
	46 PN+	2	
A?	45 AN?	–	
	47 PN?	–	–
B+	36 ON+	1	0.1
B?	37 ON?	–	–
H	48 HT	–	–
X	49 XN	4	0.3

(Excluded: $N9$, 0.8%)

Mnemonic for interpreting the combinations of letters: NS, nuclear schizophrenia; DS, schizophrenic without first rank symptoms; DP, paranoid psychosis; CS, catatonic schizophrenia; RS, residual schizophrenia; SS, simple schizophrenia; UP, XP, possible borderline psychosis; MN, mania; HM, hypomania; PD, psychotic depression; AP, affective psychosis; RD, reactive depression; ND, neurotic depression; SD, simple depression; AN, anxiety neurosis; PN, phobic neurosis; ON, obsessional neurosis; HT, hysteria; XN, residual neurosis.
These mnemonics are not to be taken seriously as 'diagnoses'.

Many of the subclasses consist of a combination of elements; for example, NSPD, DPMN, CSMN, etc. This means that two types of symptoms were predominant but the one regarded as more important in the context of the clinical picture is placed first. Thus these subclasses provide a sort of double classification and could be read as indicating a probable and a possible grouping.

8

LIMITATIONS AND USES OF THE PSE AND CATEGO SYSTEM

1. LIMITATIONS

The PSE and Catego system consists of linked components, several of which can be used independently. The advantages and disadvantages of each component therefore need separate discussion. The general limitations built into the PSE schedule have already been explained. Organic symptoms are not dealt with in any detail, although it is relatively simple to add a section to cover these and the US–UK Project has shown that such a supplement can be used reliably (J. R. M. Copeland, personal communication). Since the interview is based only on the previous month, characteristics such as personality traits or social adjustment, which require a large time period for their assessment are necessarily excluded. Separate instruments are required if such assessments are to be formalised. Previous episodes of the symptoms covered in the PSE can, however, be described by using the syndrome check list. Finally, aetiological information is not included in the PSE itself, but requires a separate schedule.

A further limitation on the use of the PSE is that ratings of symptoms made on the basis of behaviour, affect and speech observed during examination are, on the whole, less reliable than those of subjectively described symptoms. The PSE is less useful for describing characteristics which are mainly manifested in observed behaviour. This is probably due to the brief time sample available during examination which means that severe symptoms are less likely to be observed. Nurses, for example, can be trained to use behaviour rating scales, based on a week or more of observation, very reliably (Wing and Brown, 1970).

It is important to understand these limitations in order to choose the right instrument for evaluation. The PSE has certain uses, which are summarised later, and it may also be useful in conjunction with other instruments. But there are conditions for which it is not the best means of assessment.

Since the PSE and Catego system is concerned with standardising processes which every psychiatrist habitually uses, but which are not ordinarily defined very precisely, the problems which have had to be solved in order to create the system can be used to examine some of the difficulties of psychiatric description and classification. In turn, the extent to which these problems have not been solved can be used to define the limits of the system.

The first and most basic problem is to specify the criteria to be used when deciding whether a symptom is present or absent. The second, an extension of the first, is to assess clinical severity. In many cases, particularly during an acute attack of some illness, these decisions are relatively simple, because the symptom is clearly present to a severe degree. In others, the symptoms are so unlike ordinary experience and hence so rare that if they are elicited at all, they should be rated as present. Though insertion or withdrawal are of this type. Others, however, are common in mild degree and may then carry as little clinical significance as, say, a haemoglobin measurement of 90%. Anxiety and depression are of this type. Should they nevertheless be rated as present? The decision becomes of great importance in a general population survey, although in an acutely ill sample it is much easier to make because the symptoms are likely to be more severe. The rule adopted for the PSE has been that the symptom must be definitely present in order to be rated, which means that it must be clinically fairly severe. As far as possible, social factors are not taken into account in making this decision. The criteria used for neurotic symptoms are specified in the introduction to the glossary of definitions of ninth edition symptoms; the extent to which the symptom is out of voluntary control, out of proportion to circumstances and accompanied by an unpleasant affect. Each of these rules can be useful as a guide but none can be used alone. In particular, the second criterion is only useful when there is no doubt that the symptom *is* out of proportion to circumstances, for example, if worrying is out of proportion to the subject matter worried about. If the subject matter would be likely to be found severely worrying by most people this criterion cannot be used and a decision has to be made on the basis of the other two, together with the intensity, duration and frequency of the symptom. Social impairment is not taken into account in rating severity but individual factors such as degree of stoicism and culturally acceptable ways of expressing the complaint must necessarily be considered.

The limitation of the PSE data so far gathered is that the interview has mainly been used with people already referred for a psychiatric opinion. In most series they have actually been admitted to hospital. This means that they have usually been suffering from fairly definite and severe conditions. Whether the same degree of reliability of rating common symptoms such as anxiety or depression can be achieved in a general population sample has yet to be demonstrated. A screening form of the eighth edition of the PSE has been used in a pilot study with promising results and a screening version of the ninth edition is at present under test. If the same degree of reliability of symptom rating can be shown in a population sample as has been observed in samples of referred patients, it will be possible to use operational criteria for case-finding in epidemiological studies.

The third problem which had to be solved in creating the PSE and Catego system was that of differential definition of symptoms. The basic principle, incorporated into the PSE interview from the beginning, is that the examiner must be clear about the definition according to which he decides whether each symptom is present or absent and also how to distinguish one symptom from another. The structure built into the interview is subordinated to the overriding need to be sure that the subject is given every opportunity and help to describe his experiences with precision so that these clinical judgements can be made. The glossary of definitions now gives some aid both in defining each symptom and in differentiating between those which are commonly mistaken for each other. Some uncertainties still remain since some of the symptoms still overlap with each other but it may be hoped that revision based on further experience will gradually reduce these.

The fourth problem was which symptoms to include. So far as the classical symptoms are concerned the PSE schedule, even in its briefer ninth edition, is over-inclusive. Certainly far fewer symptoms are needed to make a diagnosis. (The Catego program can operate adequately on only twenty syndromes.) However, the PSE is a descriptive as well as a categorising instrument and the 140 symptoms are sufficient to cover nearly all those mentioned in current text books. However, in a different sense the list of symptoms is highly selective since data on personality characteristics such as assertiveness or amenability, and on relationships with authority figures, etc., are omitted.

The nature of the PSE is determined by these four fundamental characteristics; each of which represents a solution to a major problem arising out of the attempt to standardise clinical practice. Other systems would incorporate different methods (whether or not consciously and deliberately considered) for deciding which symptoms to include, whether they were present or not and with what degree of severity. Having established the basic check list of symptoms to be rated, another limitation on the use of the PSE is created by the technique required to conduct the interview, which is a form of 'cross-examination'. This method is necessitated by the earlier decision to specify the purpose of the interview; to rate symptoms which have already been defined in advance. The PSE is therefore neither a questionnaire nor a non-directed conversation. It is specifically directed at deciding which symptoms are present and the decision is always taken by the examiner after he has collected sufficient evidence for or against. The subject's agreement or disagreement with any particular question is not, in itself, sufficient for a decision. Subjects find the interview very acceptable and there is no need at all for any of the hectoring quality which the term 'cross-examination' may seem to imply. A skilled interviewer does not appear to be conducting a standardised interview at all. The form of the questions has been based on a long experience of how patients themselves tend to describe the symptoms, but though this experience was obtained with British patients in the first instance, the wording can be readily translated into other languages with a very different structure (see chapter 6 of volume 1 of the IPSS; WHO, 1973). It is our experience that even psychiatrists who are used to a completely non-directive technique and who do not attach great importance to the type of symptoms rated in the PSE can learn to use the interview successfully. However, a few psychiatrists are unable to do so.

The question of reliability deserves further consideration. Although the data summarised in chapter 5 indicate a satisfactory degree of reliability and repeatability in general terms, the figures quoted are fully compatible with occasional large and serious differences in the way the symptoms are understood and rated. Most of the results refer to the situation in which two psychiatrists (often two who know each other quite well) are rating one interview. The observer can pick up clues as to how the examiner proposes to rate and the reliability can thus be spuriously high. In the original MRC study (Wing *et al.*, 1967), the US–UK study (Kendell *et al.*, 1968), and the IPSS (WHO, 1973), there was a fairly extensive test of repeatability by different psychiatrists examining the same patient at intervals of a few days and the degree of agreement, though somewhat lower than in the simultaneous condition, was of much the same order. The comparisons were nearly all between psychiatrists who had been educated in the same clinical school and who knew each other well. Reliability exercises using video-taped and filmed interviews allowed some assessment of reliability between psychiatrists from different schools of thought, but it would have been of interest to assess the repeatability of the interview among psychiatrists trained in different psychiatric schools. The IPSS presented the possibility to investigate this question but language difficulties were great and such a study was not undertaken. It is possible that in spite of the fact that the PSE was used with considerable reliability within Centres there were differences between Centres in the definition and recognition of symptoms and in the technique of interviewing. Examples were given in the IPSS report (WHO, 1973) of cases where key symptoms had been rated present although the examples written down at the same time did not seem to warrant a positive rating. It is not known how often this occurred without being noted, or how often a symptom was present but not rated positively. The level of reliability that has been achieved in the assessment of video-taped interviews, however, suggests that there may not have been many major differences. The reasons for possible differences are easy to identify. Although the psychiatrists from different Centres rated patients jointly and discussed their ratings in the course of the studies, the formal training of the original group of psychiatrists was not prolonged. There was no detailed glossary of definitions of items and, in particular, no specific training in differential definition. It is well known that even an initially high reliability can deteriorate during the course of a long project. The likelihood of two or more groups of psychiatrists with different initial training and conceptions gradually deviating from each other, must also be remembered. The present manual is based upon the experience of these earlier studies and it should be possible to ensure greater uniformity in future. Meanwhile, this limitation should always be kept in mind. It applies *a fortiori* of course, to any results which are obtained by psychiatrists who have received no training at all in the use of the PSE. The training of raters is an essential part of the PSE procedure and there is no guarantee whatever that using any version of the PSE, without adequate instruction, will ensure comparability of the results with those of users who have been trained. In assessing any paper which gives results based on the use of the PSE, the reader should always take into account the training of the raters before deciding whether the data can be compared with those of the MRC, US–UK or IPSS studies.

Clearly these limitations on the use of the PSE also apply to the syndrome check list which is based on the PSE and which, in addition, has the restriction that it is not usually rated with such reliability. This applies *a fortiori* to the aetiology schedule, which is simply a method of standardising the decisions to be taken, not the methods of reaching a decision.

The results of applying the Catego procedure are limited in their interpretation not only by the restrictions already discussed in relation to the PSE which supplies the input, but also in relation to the rules of classification which are incorporated. It is clear from the evidence presented in chapter 7 that the classes do bear a close relationship to diagnoses, at least in broad terms, and that the more detailed sub-classification may also have its uses. The major limitation, however, is that the Catego classes are not intended to be regarded as a substitute for diagnosis. To take the most obvious example, only a clinician can give an opinion as to whether the symptoms rated as present, which are used to derive a classification, are likely to be worth treating. Similarly, the extent to which a patient is stuperous or incoherent or mute has to be taken into account in deciding what meaning the classification has. The combined PSE and Catego procedure produces as an end result a classification which the clinician may or may not find to be of use. That decision must itself be clinical.

Moreover, a classification of anxiety state (AN+ or PN+) could be based on a single anxiety symptom rated (1), with no social impairment rated on item 106. It is obvious enough that such a classification hardly constitutes an indication for treatment, but only à clinician is in a position to judge what it really 'means'. Operational criteria can help to set threshold definitions for case-finding in population surveys but they may mean nothing in terms of need for treatment or investigation.

The classes derived nevertheless bear an obvious resemblance to the classical system of diagnosis of 'functional' psychiatric disorders (this is particularly true of classes S, M, D, R, N, A and B) and the restriction here is that they are related mainly to that system and not, for example, to a classification in terms of unconscious processes. A good deal more work remains to be put into the addition of information from the clinical history. It is evident that the PSE contains most of the information needed for a classification but in perhaps 25% of cases data are required from records or from the present episode earlier than the preceding month. The syndrome check list is a simple way of adding this. The aetiology schedule provides a check list method of codifying the decisions necessary for converting a classification into an ICD equivalent.

The final restriction is the one discussed fully in chapter 1. The PSE and Catego procedure produces a passable imitation of diagnosis within a certain range of conditions, but the validity of the classification must depend upon external criteria. However, this limitation also introduces the uses and advantages of the system, which can be used to help investigate many different kinds of clinical problem so long as its limitations are also kept in mind.

2. USES

Paradoxically, if the procedures described in this book are used within the limits described, that is, with a proper appreciation of how they can be applied and how they cannot, the advantages of the system are likely to be maximised. Its main uses are scientific, educational and clinical.

SCIENTIFIC USES

(i) *Description of psychopathology*

The first and most obvious use of the system is to describe, in terms of symptoms, syndromes or classes, the psychopathological characteristics of groups of people at a defined point in time. Syndrome profiles (particularly of the first twenty syndromes in the SCL) are a convenient descriptive form, either for individuals or for groups. Profiles of the main Catego classes are illustrated in chapter 7. They look very similar to profiles of the equivalent diagnostic categories except that there is a higher ratio of signal to noise. Profiles using section-scores are given in publications on the US–UK study (Cooper *et al.*, 1972) and using 'units of analysis' in volume 1 of the International Pilot Study of Schizophrenia (WHO, 1973). The original paper on the PSE contained profiles of mean section scores for the diagnostic groups, neurotic depression, retarded depression, psychotic depression and anxiety state, showing marked differentiation between these categories. Four schizophrenic profiles were also illustrated (Wing *et al.*, 1967). The syndrome profiles characterising schizo-affective psychosis (manic or psychotic depressive types) were compared with those of mania and psychotic depression (Wing, 1970).

These are purely descriptive exercises, interesting because of their useful confirmation of the marked differences between classical diagnostic groupings but not otherwise particularly informative.

(ii) *Measurement of change*

An instrument which can be reliably used to produce scores representing various areas of psychopathology is likely to be valuable for measuring change. The follow-up of patients included in the IPSS series will provide an opportunity to discover how many have PSE symptoms five years after the time of initial examination and what the patterns are.

The ninth edition of the PSE has been used in two trials of preventive medication in schizophrenia. In each case, the criterion of relapse was taken as a decision by the clinician in charge to replace the trial medication (which might have been active phenothiazine or placebo) by a known phenothiazine drug. This was usually, of course, based upon his observation of a worsening of the patient's symptoms. Analysis of PSE syndrome profiles in both trials showed a marked increase in symptoms at the time of relapse; particularly in symptoms characteristic of schizophrenia, such as those in syndromes 1 (NS) and 13 (AH). Repeated PSE interviews could, in fact, have been used to help determine whether the patient had relapsed (Leff and Wing, 1971; Hirsch et al., 1973). The eighth edition of the PSE was used monthly to measure change in a trial of two anti-depressant drugs by Lipsedge, Rees and Pike (1971). Total score on neurotic symptoms and subscores on anxiety and depression all showed considerable reduction on both drugs. A self-rated scale of depression (Beck et al., 1969) was also used and the correlation with the PSE depression subscore was 0.84 (D. J. Pike, personal communication).

(iii) Standardisation of selection

One of the most important uses of the PSE and Catego system is to standardise the description of mental state of patients included in various investigations. The literature on diagnostic unreliability has been discussed in chapter 1 and though it is clear that the degree of unreliability has sometimes been exaggerated, it is also certain that many investigations suffer from the fact that their results are not strictly comparable with those undertaken elsewhere. This is particularly true, in view of the results of the US–UK and IPSS Projects, of papers published on work in parts of the United States and USSR, when compared with studies in other parts of the world. Thus the two trials of preventive medication in schizophrenia mentioned above are relevant mainly to patients with the characteristic schizophrenic symptoms included in syndromes 1 (NS) and 13 (AH). Trials which include patients with other types of 'schizophrenia', in particular the 'borderline' or 'simple' varieties, or patients with 'monosymptomatic' delusions, are to that extent non-comparable. The paper by Cole et al. (1964), for example, does not contain information which would enable a judgement to be made as to what groups of patients are included under the rubric 'schizophrenia'.

Another example may be taken from the field of family studies. Wynne and his colleagues have suggested that the parents of schizophrenic patients manifest 'communication deviances' not seen in the parents of people of similar age and social status but who do not suffer from schizophrenia (Wynne, 1968). They did not, however, give any very precise picture of the clinical condition of the patients involved and it seems probable, from the other studies mentioned earlier, that many of them would not have been diagnosed as schizophrenic in some other countries. Hirsch and Leff (1971, 1974) repeated the work but were unable to find the same marked differences between groups. Their patients were nearly all in class S according to the Catego criteria. It is at least possible that these differences are accountable in terms of a difference in diagnostic composition of the US and the UK series.

Scientific communication would be greatly facilitated if all investigations were, in future, to include a detailed statement concerning the diagnostic composition of the groups studied in such terms that other workers would be able to reproduce the same experimental conditions. Comparability in this field is vital for all scientific work.

(iv) *Investigation of taxonomic systems*

A great advantage of a system of clinical classification based upon precisely specifiable rules and closely related to a diagnostic system in wide current use, is that it offers a means of comparison with other techniques of classification, whether purely clinical as with psychiatric diagnosis or purely mathematical as with various clustering techniques. The difficulty in making comparisons with the statistical taxonomic procedures is that they have usually been used in conjunction with a numerical input which does not allow the representation of symptoms which many clinicians would regard as diagnostically important. Thus Lorr (1965), for example, has derived statistical types, in which anxiety and depression could not be separated from each other; similarly, retarded speech, retarded movement and flat affect were combined together, as were restlessness, agitation, overactivity and elation. The factor analysis by Spitzer and his colleagues (1967) gave rise to very similar results.

Fleiss, Gurland and Cooper (1971), however, using similar statistical techniques based upon an input derived from PSE ratings, found that phobic anxiety could be distinguished from depression, retarded speech from retarded movement and flat affect from both, and restlessness from manic symptoms. These discriminations were important for the differential diagnosis between mania, anxiety states, depression, and subgroups of schizophrenia. The authors conclude, unsurprisingly, that output depends upon input. Clinically rich procedures such as the PSE, quite apart from the advantages derived from standard definitions of symptoms and partial standardisation of the interview technique, are likely to give rise to a larger number of factors, clusters or types when subjected to statistical analysis. These clusters are also likely to be closer to the diagnostic categories used by clinical psychiatrists who take diagnosis seriously. The upshot of these comparisons is that the results of factor and cluster analyses cannot be compared if they are based on markedly dissimilar inputs.

If the principles incorporated in the Catego program are indeed similar to those adopted by diagnosticians, it is evident that there is another very fundamental difference between statistical and clinical methods of allocating cases to categories. This is that clinical diagnosis is hierarchical. If organic symptoms such as disorientation or loss of memory or epilepsy are present, other symptoms are regarded as of less diagnostic importance. In fact, practically any other symptom can be present, including first rank symptoms of schizophrenia, elation, depression, obsessions, anxiety or hysterical conversion symptoms, without being regarded as having diagnostic value in themselves. If there are no organic phenomena, the symptoms with the highest diagnostic significance are the first rank schizophrenic symptoms.

Again, any other symptoms lower in the hierarchy may be present, but they can only somewhat modify the diagnosis (e.g. help in subclassification); they cannot determine it. Although the principle becomes less clear in the lower reaches of the diagnostic hierarchy it can still be discerned and specified. It is built into the entire range of Catego decisions.

Nearly all statistical studies ignore the hierarchical principle, since they are built upon the premise that every input datum must be given the same weight as every other. From a clinical point of view this assumption is nonsensical, not least because it is evident that many symptoms depend upon the presence of others. For example, in clinical terms, an individual may worry because he has something to worry about, because he is a worrier, because he has phobias, because he has depressive preoccupations, because he has persecutory delusions, because he has first rank symptoms, or because he has noticed that his memory is failing. To give the symptom 'worrying' the same weight diagnostically as any of the others makes no clinical sense at all.

Kendell (1973) has shown that reasonable diagnoses can be made after reading transcripts of five-minute interviews with acutely-ill patients concerning their main symptoms, in response to questions about why they were coming into hospital, what had been going wrong recently and whether they regarded themselves as ill. If the hierarchical principle is correct, all that need be known in many cases are the highly discriminating symptoms at each level of the diagnostic hierarchy. Kendell's data suggest that this is true of some three-quarters of admitted patients. The data presented in chapter 7, particularly in tables 7.7, 7.8 and 7.15, tend towards a similar conclusion.

Further examples of the use of the Catego procedure to throw light on the processes of clinical diagnosis may be found in chapter 7 and in volume 1 of the IPSS project. Many of the questions raised are concerned directly or indirectly with the question of validity. It was one of the main purposes of developing the PSE and Catego system that studies of such questions should be facilitated. So far, they have only been used indirectly in studies of the treatment and prognosis of schizophrenia, in which it was shown that patients in class S, whose characteristic symptoms had mainly been controlled by medication with phenothiazine drugs, experienced in a large proportion of cases a recrudescence of symptoms from the (NS) and (AH) syndromes when medication was withdrawn at random and a placebo substituted (Leff and Wing, 1971; Hirsch et al., 1973). The categorisation at the time of relapse was nearly always the same (i.e. class S) as during the previous acute episode, during which the patients had been selected for the trial. Findings of this kind lend a certain solidity to the concept of schizophrenia represented by Catego class S and give legitimate reason for hope that other investigations using the PSE and Catego system will help to refine and improve some of the disease theories in current use. Classes P and O, however, probably include many different subgroups, some of which may not best be explained in terms of disease theories.

USES FOR TEACHING

Because the ninth edition of the PSE and the associated computer classification program are rather more systematic, standardised, reliable and precise than ordinary clinical practice, and because they are based on a specifiable set of definitions and rules, they may be found a useful teaching aid in those schools where the equivalent clinical system is already being taught. Because the whole system is equivalent to a brief text book of psychopathology couched in operational terms, the experienced clinical teacher can be clear as to which definitions, procedures or decisions he does not accept and can specify his alternative rules. He can also compare the results of a young clinician with his own, either during live interviews or using filmed or taped records. Discussions of any differences can be highly informative to all parties, both in illuminating the technical problems of diagnostic interviewing and in bringing to light differences in how symptoms or syndromes or diagnostic classes are defined. The results can also be used to improve the standard system. The authors would be very grateful for suggestions for changing the PSE schedule, the glossary of definitions or the Catego program, since they have no doubt that there are still many places where definitions are vague or contradictory, where symptoms are redundant or have been omitted incorrectly, and where decision claims could be made more efficient or more clinically relevant.

CLINICAL USES

Insofar as the system is simply a standardisation of an ordinary clinical approach, a psychiatrist could incorporate it into his everyday work. Many of those using it have found that their style of interviewing, coverage and ability to describe psychopathology improve. However, all clinical decisions are the responsibility of the psychiatrist, and not of any particular instrument or aid which he happens to be using. In the last resort, the decision as to whether to pursue a particular line of questioning, whether to accept a patient's description as evidence for the presence of a symptom or whether to conclude that he is mimicking or faking (Rosenhan, 1973), and whether to make use of a computer categorisation, can only be taken by the psychiatrist himself.

This is a good point at which to end this manual since, although our immediate purpose has been scientific, our long-term goal is to contribute, even if indirectly, to that progressive development in clinical medicine which has resulted in the reduction of much human suffering and in the prevention of much functional impairment. We should like to think that the use of the techniques described in this book would make the clinical process more effective and more useful.

REFERENCES

Beck A. T., Ward C. H., Mendelson M., Mock J. and Erbaugh J. (1961). An inventory for measuring depression. *Arch. gen. Psychiat.* **4**, 561–71.

Beck A. T., Ward C. H., Mendelson M., Mock J. and Erbaugh J. (1962). Reliability of psychiatric diagnoses: a study of consistency of clinical judgements and ratings. *Amer. J. Psychiat.* **119**, 351–7.

Binitie A. A. O. (1971). *A Study of Depression in Benin, Nigeria*. M.D. Thesis, London University.

Birnbaum A. and Maxwell A. E. (1961). Classification procedures based on Bayes's formula. *Applied Statistics* **9**, 152–69.

Brown G. W., Birley J. L. T. and Wing J. K. (1972). Influence of family life on the course of schizophrenic disorders: a replication. *Brit. J. Psychiat.* **121**, 241–58.

Cohen J. (1968). Weighted kappa: nominal scale agreement with provision for sealed disagreement or partial credit. *Psychol. Bull.* **70**, 213–20.

Cole J. O. *et al.* (1964). Phenothiazine treatment in acute schizophrenia. *Arch. gen. Psychiat.* **10**, 246–61.

Cooper J. E., Kendell R. E., Gurland B. J., Sharpe L., Copeland J. R. M. and Simon R. (1972). *Psychiatric Diagnosis in New York and London*. London: Oxford University Press.

Cranach M. von and Cooper J. E. (1972). Changes in rating behaviour during the learning of a standardized psychiatric interview. *Psychol. Med.* **2**, 373–80.

Edwards D. A. W. (1971). Discriminative information in diagnosis. *Proceedings of the Royal Society of Medicine* **64**, 676.

Endicott J. and Spitzer R. L. (1972). What! Another rating scale: the psychiatric evaluation form. *J. nerv. men. Dis.* **154**, 88–104.

Endicott J. and Spitzer R. L. (1973). Current and past psychopathology scales (CAPPS): rationale, reliability and validity. *Arch. gen. Psychiat.*

Everitt B. S., Gourlay A. J. and Kendell R. E. (1971). An attempt at validation of traditional psychiatric syndromes by cluster analysis. *Brit. J. Psychiat.* **119**, 399–412.

Fischer M. (1973). Development and validity of a computerised method for diagnosis of functional psychoses (Diax). To be published.

Fleiss J. L., Gurland B. J. and Cooper J. E. (1971). Some contributions to the measurement of psychopathology. *Brit. J. Psychiat.* **119**, 647–56.

Fleiss J. L., Spitzer R., Cohen J. and Endicott J. (1974). Three computer diagnosis methods compared. To be published.

Foulds G. A. (1965). *Personality and Personal Illness*. London: Tavistock.

General Register Office (1968). *A Glossary of Mental Disorders*. London: HMSO.

Gleisner J., Hewett S. and Mann S. (1972). Reasons for admission to hospital. In: Wing J. K. and Hailey A. M. (eds.) *Evaluating a Community Psychiatric Service*. London: Oxford University Press.

138   REFERENCES

Goldberg D., Cooper B., Eastwood M. R., Kedward H. B., Shepherd M. (1970). Standardised psychiatric interview for use in community surveys. *Brit. J. Prev. Soc. Med.* **24**, 18.

Grosz H. J. and Grossman K. G. (1968). Clinicians' response style: a source of variation and bias in clinical judgements. *J. Abnorm. Psychol.* **73**, 207–14.

Hamilton M. (1960). A rating scale for depression. *J. Neurol. Neurosurg. Psychiat.* **23**, 56–62.

Hays W. L. (1967). *Statistics for Psychologists*. New York: Brooks-Cole.

Hempel C. G. (1959). Introduction to problems of taxonomy. In: Zubin J. (ed.) *Field Studies in the Mental Disorders*. New York: Grune and Stratton.

Hirsch S. R., Gaind R., Rohde P. D., Stevens B. C. and Wing J. K. (1973). Outpatient maintenance of chronic schizophrenic patients with long-acting fluphenazone: double-blind placebo trial. *Brit. med. J.* **1**, 633–7.

Hirsch S. R. and Leff J. P. (1971). Parental abnormalities of verbal communication in the transmission of schizophrenia. *Psychol. Med.* **1**, 118–27.

Hirsch S. R. and Leff J. P. (1974). *Abnormality in Parents of Schizophrenics: A Review of the Literature and an Investigation of Communication Defects and Deviances*. London: Oxford University Press.

Itard J. M. G. (1932). *The Wild Boy of Aveyron* (trans. Humphrey G. and Humphrey M.). New York: Appleton-Century-Crofts.

Kanner L. (1943). Autistic disturbances of affective contact. *Nervous Child* **2**, 217–50.

Kendell R. E. (1973). Psychiatric diagnoses: a study of how they are made. *Brit. J. Psychiat.* **122**, 437–45.

Kendell R. E., Everitt B., Cooper J. E., Sartorius N. and David M. E. (1968). Reliability of the Present State Examination. *Social Psychiatry* **3**, 123–9.

Kreitman N. (1961). Reliability of psychiatric diagnosis. *Journal of Mental Science* **107**, 876.

Kreitman N., Sainsbury P., Morrissey J., Towers J. and Scrivener J. (1961). Reliability of psychiatric assessment: an analysis. *Journal of Mental Science* **107**, 887.

Leff J. P. and Vaughn C. (1972). Psychiatric patients in-contact and out-of-contact with services: a clinical and social assessment. In Wing J. K. and Hailey A. M. (eds.) *Evaluating a Community Psychiatric Service*. London: Oxford University Press.

Leff J. P. and Wing J. K. (1971). Trial of maintenance therapy in schizophrenia. *Brit. med. J.* **3**, 599–604.

Lipsedge M. S., Rees W. L. and Pike D. J. (1971). A double-blind comparison of Dothiepin and Amitriptyline for the treatment of depression with anxiety. *Psychopharmacologia* (Berl.) **19**, 153–62.

Lorr M. (1965). A typology for functional psychotics. In Katz M. M., Cole J. O. and Barton W. E. (eds.) *Classification in Psychiatry and Psychopathology*. Chevy Chase, Md: NIMH.

Lorr M. (ed.) (1966). *Explorations in typing psychotics*. London and New York: Pergamon.

Lorr M., Klett C. J. and McNair D. M. (1963). *Syndromes of Psychosis*. New York: MacMillan.

Lorr M., Klett C. J., McNair D. M. and Lasky J. (1963). *In-patient Multidimensional Psychiatric Scale* (Manual). Palo Alto: Consulting Psychologists Press.

Mann S. and Sproule J. (1972). Reasons for a six-month stay. In Wing J. K. and Hailey A. M. (eds.) *Evaluating a Community Psychiatric Service*. London: Oxford University Press.

Maxwell A. E. (1970). Comparing the classification of subjects by two independent judges. *Brit. J. Psychiat.* **116**, 651–5.

Meehl P. E. and Rosen A. (1955). Antecedent probability and the efficiency of psychometric signs, patterns or cutting scores. *Psychol Bull.* **52**, 194–216.

Overall J. E. and Gorham D. R. (1962). The brief psychiatric rating scale. *Psychol. Rep.* **10**, 799–812.

Roe A. (1949). Clinical practice and personality theory: a symposium. IV, Integration of personality theory and clinical practice. *J. abnorm. soc. Psychol.* **44**, 36.

Rosenhan D. L. (1973). On being sane in insane places. *Science* **179**, 250–8.

Sartorius N., Brooke E. and Lin T. Y. (1970). Reliability of psychiatric assessment in international research. In: Hare E. H. and Wing J. K. (eds.) *Psychiatric Epidemiology.* London: Oxford University Press.

Scharfetter C. (1971). *Das AMP-System: Manual zur Dokumentation psychiatrischer Befunde.* Heidelberg: Springer Verlag.

Schmidt H. O. and Fonda C. P. (1956). The reliability of psychiatric diagnosis: a new look. *J. abnorm. soc. Psychol.* **52**, 262.

Schneider K. (1959). *Clinical Psychopathology* (trans. Hamilton M. W.). London and New York: Grune and Stratton.

Schneider K. (1971). *Klinische Psychopathologie* (9th ed.). Stuttgart: Thieme.

Simon R. J., Gurland B. J., Fleiss J. L. and Sharpe L. (1971). Impact of a patient history interview on psychiatric diagnosis. *Arch. gen. Psychiat.* **24**, 437–40.

Spitzer R. and Endicott J. (1968). DIAGNO: A computer program for psychiatric diagnosis utilizing the differential diagnostic procedure. *Arch. gen. Psychiat.* **18**, 746–56.

Spitzer R. L. and Endicott J. (1969). DIAGNO II: further developments in a computer program for psychiatric diagnosis. *American Journal of Psychiatry* **125**, Suppl. 12–21.

Spitzer R. L., Endicott J. and Cohen J. (1967). Mental status schedule: proportion of factor analytically derived scales. *Archives of General Psychiatry* **16**, 479.

Spitzer R. L., Endicott J. and Fleiss J. L. (1967). Instruments and recording forms for evaluating psychiatric states and history. *Comprehensive Psychiatry* **8**, 321.

Spitzer R. L., Endicott J., Fleiss J. L. and Cohen J. (1970). The Psychiatric Status Schedule: a technique for evaluating psychopathology and impairment in role functioning. *Arch. gen. Psychiat.* **23**, 41–55.

Spitzer R. L., Fleiss J. L., Burdock E. I. and Hardesty A. S. (1964). The mental status schedule: rationale, reliability and validity. *Comprehensive Psychiatry* **5**, 384–95.

Taylor J. A. (1953). A personality scale of manifest anxiety. *J. abn. soc. Psychol.* **48**, 285–90.

Wing J. K. (1970). A standard form of psychiatric present state examination (PSE) and a method for standardising the classification of symptoms. In: Hare E. H. and Wing J. K. (eds.) *Psychiatric Epidemiology: An International Symposium.* London: Oxford University Press.

Wing J. K. (1971). Standardisation of psychiatric classification. *Proceedings of the Royal Society of Medicine* **64**, 673–5.

Wing J. K. (1974). Schizophrenia: medical and social models. To be published.

Wing J. K., Birley J. L. T., Cooper J. E., Graham P. and Isaacs A. (1967). Reliability of a procedure for measuring and classifying 'present psychiatric state'. *Brit. J. Psychiat.* **113**, 499–515.

140   REFERENCES

Wing J. K. and Brown G. W. (1970). *Institutionalism and Schizophrenia.* London: Cambridge University Press.

Wing L., Wing J. K., Griffiths D. and Stevens B. (1972). An epidemiological and experimental evaluation of industrial rehabilitation of chronic psychotic patients in the community. In: Wing J. K. and Hailey A. M. (eds.) *Evaluating a Communi Psychiatric Service.* London: Oxford University Press.

Wittenborn J. R. (1951). Symptom patterns in a group of mental hospital patients. *J. consulting Psychol.* **15**, 290–302.

Wittenborn J. R. (1955). *Wittenborn Psychiatric Rating Scales.* New York: Psychological Corporation.

World Health Organisation (1973). *The International Pilot Study of Schizophrenia.* Geneva: WHO.

Wynne L. C. (1968). Methodologic and conceptual issues in the study of schizophrenics and their families. In: Rosenthal D. and Kety S. S. (eds.) *The Transmission of Schizophrenia.* New York: Pergamon.

Zubin J. (1967). Classification of the behaviour disorders. *Ann. Rev. Psychol.* **18**, 373–401.

GLOSSARY OF DEFINITIONS OF SYMPTOMS INCLUDED IN THE NINTH EDITION OF THE PSE

SCORING

There are two major decision points in the (0), (1), (2) scoring system used for nearly all the 140 symptoms. The first is whether or not the symptom is present; i.e. whether the rating should be (0), or either (1) or (2). The second is whether it is present in moderate or severe form; i.e. whether the rating should be (1) or (2). In the last resort, such decisions are clinical and will be based on a judgement of many interacting factors.

Certain operational principles can be laid down, but none is absolute. However, if used in combination they will be found useful guides to clinical judgement.

The terms 'psychotic', 'borderline' and 'non-psychotic' are very variably defined. An arbitrary criterion could be applied: most of the symptoms in sections 2–11 being called 'neurotic' with a few 'borderline'; section 12 being 'borderline' and sections 13–15 'psychotic'. Sections 18, 19 and 20 could be similarly partitioned. However this would be likely to cause misunderstanding, since it is difficult for readers to remember that no theoretical assumptions are intended when such operationally defined labels are applied. Section numbers will therefore usually be used instead. However, it is useful to be able to use a short-hand term like 'psychotic' rather than always to have to refer to 'symptoms in sections 13–15' (a phrase which has no convenient adjectival form). It must be emphasised that this usage has no theoretical significance.

No distinction is made between symptoms (e.g. subjectively experienced anxiety) and signs (e.g. an anxious facies, tremor of the hands, sweating palms, etc.). Both are discussed, for convenience, as symptoms.

The code (8) is used for 'not known'. This means that the examiner is not sure whether the symptom has been present during the past month, even though the appropriate questions have been asked, and answered without incoherence or evasion. The symptom cannot be excluded.

The code (9) is used for 'not applicable'. This means that no rating can be made because the questions were not asked or the subject does not answer, or the answer is incomprehensible.

DIFFERENTIATION BETWEEN PRESENCE OR ABSENCE OF SYMPTOMS (SECTIONS 2-11)

Obviously the main criterion is whether the subject describes the symptom as defined in the glossary. However, the threshold between 'present' and 'absent' may be difficult to define and three rules will be found useful as guides to a decision.

(a) The symptom is beyond conscious control. For example, the subject cannot stop worrying, cannot resist an obsessional idea or cannot cut short a panic attack even though he tries to and takes much thought about it. Another way of judging is according to whether other people can distract the subject from his worries or his depression or anxiety or whether he can manage this by himself, e.g. by working harder, or taking up some activity which is usually interesting, or deliberately turning attention from the symptom to something else.

(b) The symptom is out of proportion to the circumstances. This criterion is useful when there are few obvious environmental problems or if the subject is worrying about something trivial. If there are serious environmental problems such as poor housing, a tense marriage, a handicapped child in the family, financial difficulties, etc., this criterion is not so useful, and the other two criteria must be used to establish whether the symptom is present or not. A clinical judgement has to be made about the relevance of any subcultural component in reaction to external events.

(c) The symptom is accompanied by an unpleasant affect. In a very chronic condition, the affective component may become blunted. For example, the struggle against obsessional ideas may become much less marked even though the symptom is still definitely present. It is best not to use this criterion in a long-standing condition. Clearly this criterion may also fail to apply when the subject is in a euphoric or elated mood, although this quite often does have an unpleasant quality to it. Finally, the clinician has to make some judgement concerning the degree to which the subject tends to complain about subjective experiences. Some patients tend to under report the severity of a symptom, others to exaggerate. A clinical judgement has to be made also about the relevance of any variations.

RATINGS OF SEVERITY OF SYMPTOMS IN SECTIONS 2-11

Most of the points in the following paragraphs are explained in the schedule alongside each item, but they are brought together here so as to illustrate the principles of scoring which have developed during the various editions of the PSE.

Once it has been decided that a 'neurotic' symptom is present, the scoring of severity, i.e. a decision as between a rating of (1) or (2), depends upon several factors. The examiner should rate on the basis of clinical severity, that is, on the frequency and intensity of the symptom. Degree of social impairment (e.g. time off work or interference with social relationships) is rated in section 17 of the ninth edition schedule and, so far as possible, should not be used as a criterion of clinical severity. The same is true of subjective distress which is not necessarily a measure of clinical severity. In some instances the subject may not be able to distinguish between the various forms of severity, in which case the examiner may be forced to estimate the degree of clinical severity from the degree of social impairment or personal distress. Allowance should then be made, so far as possible, for the patient's social circumstances (e.g. he may be able to cover up a severe impairment if the work or family situation is protective) and for his degree of stoicism.

In most cases, clinical severity is a continuous variable, but the lower limit is fairly well recognisable from the definition. The symptom should not be rated as present unless clearly recognised; otherwise use 'not sure' (8) or (0). A rating of (1) means that it was definitely present in moderate degree sometime during the month or, if severe, was not predominant (roughly speaking, not present as much as 50% of the time). If present in severe form for more than 50% of the time, rate (2). That is, (2) means *really* severe.

For certain symptoms, such as panic attacks, it is convenient to define severity more specifically in terms of frequency. Uncommon symptoms (e.g. subjective ideomotor pressure and depersonalisation), need special rules.

Instructions are given in the PSE schedule itself concerning each individual symptom.

SCORING OF SYMPTOMS IN SECTIONS 12-15

The scoring of (1) and (2) is different for symptoms in sections 12-15 since it is usually difficult to decide how much of the time a subject is preoccupied with the abnormal experiences.

In section 12, on perceptual disorders other than hallucinations or depersonalisation, the symptoms are so rare that (2) is scored if the experience has been present at all during the month; (1) is used if the examiner considers it likely to have been present, even though the subject has not described it precisely. Delusional elaborations are not scored in this section, but under the appropriate delusion.

In section 13, on thought echo, etc. (1) and (2) are differentiated according to whether the experience is localised within the subject's own mind; e.g. if there is pure thought echo or the subject's own unconscious thoughts are supposed to be responsible, the rating is (1). If the experience is regarded as originating outside the patient's own mind, it is rated (2).

In sections 12 and 13, there are two exceptions to these rules: symptoms (49), 'unfamiliarity and delusional mood', and (59) 'thoughts being read'. These are dealt with in the same way as delusional symptoms in section 15.

In section 14, on hallucinations, (1) and (2) are used in similar ways to those described above, according to the symptom involved. Instructions for each symptom are given in the text.

The general rule for section 15, on delusions, is that a rating of (1) is reserved for 'partial' delusions, which are expressed with doubt or as possibilities which the patient entertains but is not certain about. If there is evidence that full delusional conviction has occurred during the month, even if only briefly, the rating should be (2).

RATING OF BEHAVIOUR, SPEECH AND AFFECT

Behaviour, speech and affect are rated in sections 18, 19 and 20, on the basis of observations during the examination only. A rating of (1) is reserved for a moderate or intermittent disorder, while (2) is rated for severe or fairly continuous disorder.

DEFINITIONS OF SYMPTOMS AND CRITERIA FOR RATING

1. SUBJECTIVE EVALUATION OF PHYSICAL HEALTH

This estimate should be made irrespective of the actual condition of the subject's health during the past month. Distinguish between a positive statement of fitness or health (0) and a statement only that the patient does not feel unwell (1). If the subject does feel unwell, rate according to his subjective estimate of incapacity – moderate (2) or severe (3).

2. PRESENCE OF PHYSICAL ILLNESS OR HANDICAP

This is an estimate of the subject's actual physical condition during the past month. Take into account all the information available including the results of recent investigations and examinations. If no significant illness or handicap present, rate (0). If mild but significant illness or handicap (e.g. influenza or limp), rate (1). If there is some more serious illness or handicap but it is not incapacitating or threatening to life (e.g. deafness or duodenal ulcer), rate (2). If it is severely handicapping or threatening (e.g. blindness or carcinoma), rate (3). Specify the type of illness, the disability it causes and the duration.

3. PRESENCE OF PSYCHOSOMATIC SYMPTOMS

A separate list of psychosomatic items is included which can be used or not, as desired. If any item on the list is scored (2), this is recorded as (2) in the box. If there is no rating of (2), but any item is rated (1), record as (1) in the box. If there is no positive rating on any item, record as (0).

4. WORRYING

This is perhaps the most ubiquitous psychiatric symptom and has no diagnostic significance. Regardless of content, the following three characteristics must *all* be present, otherwise the symptom is rated absent:
(i)   a round of painful, unpleasant or uncomfortable thought
(ii) which cannot be stopped voluntarily
(iii) and which is out of proportion to the subject worried about.

The subject's own mental state may be a subject of worry; he may worry about his lack of energy or social inadequacy or psychotic experiences. He can overreact to some serious matter such as the death of a near relative, or be consumed with worry about a triviality.

The numerical rating requires the examiner's judgement as to how severe and how prolonged the worrying has been during the past month.

5. TENSION PAINS

This symptom arises out of 'muscular tension' (symptom no. 7) but is localised to certain muscle groups. One of the commonest complaints is of a 'band round the temples' or 'a weight pressing down on the head', due to tension in the muscles of the scalp. Differentiate from other causes of headache (which should *not* be rated under this heading). Write down the localisation of the tension pains whenever this symptom is rated as present. Other common localisations are the back, the neck and the shoulders. Chest pain may also be due to muscular tension. If there is any doubt about a specific organic cause for the pain, rate 8 (if not known) or 9 (if pains thought to have specific cause).

Rate severity on the basis of intensity and frequency during past month.

6. TIREDNESS

This symptom often accompanies symptoms such as 'muscular tension' (no. 7), 'restlessness' (no. 8) and 'worrying' (no. 4) but it should be rated independently. The same three criteria as for 'worrying' (symptom no. 4) should be used: the subject experiences the tiredness as unpleasant, he is unable voluntarily to overcome it and it is inappropriate to the situation he finds himself in. Thus tiredness at the end of a hard day's work, or due to the after-effect of influenza, would not count.

The most intense form of the symptom is exhaustion. Rate on the basis of frequency and intensity during the past month.

7. MUSCULAR TENSION

This symptom has the same components as worrying (see symptom no. 4). The subject feels an unpleasant tension in one or more groups of muscles, he is unable to relax them when he wishes to do so, and the muscular tension is unrelated to any specific muscular effort he wishes to make.

Almost any group of muscles can be specifically affected (see symptom no. 5) but in the present symptom only general tension is rated. Rate on the basis of frequency and intensity during the past month.

Be careful to differentiate *muscular* tension from *nervous* tension. The two often go together but they are different symptoms. Nervous tension is a subjective feeling of inner restlessness or being 'keyed up' and is not defined in terms of muscular reactions at all.

8. RESTLESSNESS AND FIDGETING

This symptom is muscular tension (symptom no. 7) expressed in motor activity. In moderate degree it is shown by fidgeting of various parts of the body and an inability to stay still. In severe degree it is expressed by pacing up and down, wandering about, inability to sit down for very long. The same criteria as for 'worrying' (symptom no. 4) must be used – the restlessness is experienced as unpleasant, it is not under voluntary control and it is inappropriate to the situation the patient finds himself in.

The rating of severity is based on the subject's account of frequency and intensity during the past month. If present during the interview in marked degree, it is rated as 'agitation' (symptom no. 111).

9. HYPOCHONDRIASIS

Hypochondriasis has all the characteristics of worrying (see symptom no. 4) but the worrying is specifically concentrated on the possibility of disease or malfunction in the subject. The worrying must be painful or unpleasant, it must be beyond the subject's power to control and it must be out of proportion to any degree of illness or malfunctioning that is present.

If there is a distinct possibility that the subject has a serious disease, rate (9).

If the subject frequently and spontaneously during the interview reverts to a hypochondriacal preoccupation, rate (2). Any other degree of preoccupation during the past month, if the examiner is satisfied that the symptom has been present at all, is rated (1).

Any delusional elaboration or interpretation is *not* rated within this symptom, but rated as hypochondriacal delusions (symptom no. 91).

10. NERVOUS TENSION

Many subjects complain of a feeling of 'nervousness', 'nervous tension', 'being on edge', 'being keyed up', etc. 'Muscular tension' (symptom no. 7) is frequently present but it is not the same symptom and should be rated independently. 'Nervous tension' is differentiated from 'anxiety' (symptom no. 11) by the fact that it is not necessary for clear-cut autonomic accompaniments to be present.

'Nervous tension' has the same three components as 'worrying' (symptom no. 4) – it is unpleasant, it is not under voluntary control, and it is out of proportion to the situation the subject finds himself in. Being keyed up before taking an examination, for example, is *not* the symptom.

Rate according to the intensity and frequency of the symptom described by the subject during the past month.

11. FREE-FLOATING AUTONOMIC ANXIETY

The essential requirement for a rating of this symptom is clear-cut automatic reaction such as palpitations, difficulty getting breath, etc. (see check list in PSE), accompanied by an affect of fear or apprehension. Other unpleasant affects (e.g. nervous tension or depression) are not included in the rating: provision is made for rating them elsewhere (e.g. symptoms no. 10 and 23) and it is important to keep them separate. Similarly, isolated autonomic symptoms such as occasional palpitations, in the absence of the affect of anxiety, are not included in this symptom. The autonomic anxiety should be free-floating, that is, not exclusively tied to some particular situation. A very common occasion is when the subject is trying to go off to sleep, and with his ear pressed into the pillow, hears his heart beating. A minor change in rhythm may make him think his heart will stop and the autonomic reaction may then escalate. A subjective feeling that he is unable to take a breath properly is another common occurrence. If such reactions are confined to certain situations they should be rated under 'situational anxiety', 'anxiety on meeting people' or 'specific anxiety' (symptoms no. 15, 16 or 17). Do not include anxious foreboding as defined in symptom no. 12 below.

Do not, of course, include anxiety appropriate to the situation, e.g. going into battle, narrowly avoiding a traffic accident, realistic fear of punishment, anxiety during an examination, etc.

Anxiety due to delusions, e.g. that the subject is being hunted and may be killed, should *not* be included but rated separately (symptom no. 13). Rate (9) on present symptom if no. 13 cannot be distinguished from it.

Severity is rated according to intensity and frequency during the past month.

Always write down the autonomic reaction which the patient shows.

12. ANXIOUS FOREBODING WITH AUTONOMIC ACCOMPANIMENTS

The subject feels anxious but this is due to a feeling that something terrible is going to happen (death, disaster, ruination). It may occur in particularly concentrated form first thing in the morning, when the subject feels that he is unable to face the day ahead and experiences autonomic symptoms as he thinks about it. Do not include simple free-floating anxiety unaccompanied by this feeling, or caused by a sudden apprehension that the subject's heart will stop, etc. (this is rated in symptom no. 11 above). Severity is rated according to intensity and frequency during the month.

13. ANXIETY DUE TO DELUSIONS

The criteria for autonomic anxiety given for symptom no. 11 should be present but the cause is a delusional belief or experience. For example, the subject may hear a voice saying that he is to be killed or may experience a sensation which he believes is due to some harmful influence. From the subject's point of view such anxiety is realistic and it should not be included under symptom no. 11. Not all patients with such experiences feel any anxiety and specific enquiry must be made.

14. PANIC ATTACKS

Panic attacks are discrete episodes of autonomic anxiety, defined as for symptom no. 11, which the subject tries to terminate by taking some drastic avoiding action. The subject who cannot get his breath may rush outside for air, the subject with a phobia of travelling may have to leave the bus, the subject who is anxious when left alone may telephone her husband or go into a neighbour's house. Both free-floating and situational forms of anxiety may give rise to panic attacks. If so both should be included in the rating. Panic attacks due to delusions are not included.

Severity is rated solely in terms of frequency.

Always write down an example of any panic attack that has occurred during the month.

15. SITUATIONAL AUTONOMIC ANXIETY

This symptom consists of autonomic anxiety (defined as for symptom no. 11) which is confined to certain environments. Examples are autonomic anxiety due to being alone, to being in a confined or open space (buses, lifts, trains, cars, fields, squares, heights, etc.), to being in crowds, to crossing a busy road, etc. See check list in PSE text. Panic attacks may occur and should be included in the rating.

Two types of situation are *not* included but rated separately. The first is autonomic anxiety occurring when the subject meets people (symptom no. 16). The second is autonomic anxiety due to very specific causes, such as fear of feathers, birds, spiders, insects, cats, etc. (symptom no. 17). These two symptoms may, of course, co-exist with 'situational anxiety' and then more than one rating will be necessary. Similarly, subjects may suffer from both 'free-floating autonomic anxiety' (symptom no. 11) and 'situational anxiety', and both symptoms will then be rated as present.

The rating of severity depends on whether the subject has been in an anxiety-provoking situation during the past month. If he has not, but knows that anxiety would have occurred if he had, rate (1). If he has been in the situation, and *was* anxious according to the definition, even if on only one occasion, rate (2).

Always write down examples of the situations in which a subject becomes anxious and how the patient copes with them.

16. AUTONOMIC ANXIETY ON MEETING PEOPLE

The criteria for autonomic anxiety are those discussed for 'free-floating autonomic anxiety' (symptom no. 11). The autonomic anxiety occurs specifically in situations where the subject has to meet other people (usually strangers or acquaintances). Other 'situational anxiety' or 'specific phobias' (symptoms no. 15 and 17) may also be present in the same subject, but it is important to differentiate this particular symptom since it can occur alone.

If the subject has not been in such a situation during the past month, but recognises that he would have been anxious if the situation had occurred, rate (1). If the subject has been anxious according to the criteria laid down, when meeting other people during the past month, rate (2) even if this only occurred once. Write down an account of the circumstances.

17. SPECIFIC PHOBIAS

Autonomic anxiety, of the kind described for symptom no. 11 must have been present but the cause is a specific and limited one, e.g. mice, insects, snakes, cats, feathers, birds, etc. See check list in text of PSE. The anxiety may generalise – e.g. the subject may be unable to leave the house for fear of meeting a cat. In that case rate both 'situational anxiety' (symptom no. 15) and 'specific phobia' as present. 'Free-floating autonomic anxiety' (symptom no. 11) may also be present in which case it is rated in addition.

If the situation has not occurred during the past month but the subject is aware that he would have been anxious if it had, rate (1). If the situation has occurred and the subject was anxious according to the definition, even on only one occasion, rate (2).

18. AVOIDANCE OF AUTONOMIC ANXIETY

Use the definition of autonomic anxiety given for symptom no. 11. Anxiety may be avoided by not entering into situations known to provoke it and subjects may adopt routines which enable them to avoid anxiety altogether. Avoidance procedures may generalise until the subject is quite unable to leave the house.

Do not rate this symptom as present unless you are quite satisfied that the patient was avoiding a situation in which he had at some time (not necessarily during the past month) been autonomically anxious. Simply living a restricted life is not sufficient evidence. On the other hand, the extent of the avoidance may sometimes not be clear to the subject, so that careful questioning may be necessary to elucidate the matter.

Rate severity according to the extent of generalisation of avoidance. Rate (2), for example, if subject has been confined to the house for as long as a few days, or has been able to leave only if accompanied. Remember that there may be many techniques of avoidance without the subject becoming housebound (moving house so as to be able to walk to work rather than taking a bus, etc.).

Write down an example of any avoidance mechanism found to be present.

19. INEFFICIENT THINKING

The subject complains that he is unable to think clearly or efficiently or to reach decisions easily even about simple matters. His thoughts are muddled or slow and they tend to go round and round in aimless circles. This complaint is subjective and may be in contrast to the clear and efficient way in which the subject describes the symptom. Only the subjective complaint is rated. However, the following three criteria must always apply: the experience is unpleasant, it does not respond to the subject's voluntary attempts to end it, and it is out of proportion to the difficulties of the problems being considered.

If thought insertion, commentary, withdrawal or broadcast (symptoms no. 55-58), or any kind of delusional explanation for thought disorder are present, rate (9).

Some subjects may complain that their thought processes have always been muddled, throughout their lives. Rate complaints concerning the past month, irrespective of the previous history.

Rate severity according to frequency and intensity during the past month.

20. POOR CONCENTRATION

The subject complains that he cannot give his full attention to matters which require it or not for as long as they require. The experience is unpleasant, it is beyond the subject's power to correct except for very brief intervals, and it is out of proportion to the difficulty of the problems being considered. At its most intense, the subject cannot even read a few sentences in a newspaper, cannot watch television and cannot take in a conversation. Severity is rated on the basis of frequency and intensity during the past month.

If a subject has thought insertion, commentary, withdrawal or broadcast (symptoms no. 55-58), or any kind of delusional explanation for thought disorder, rate (9).

There may be several other reasons for poor concentration, including worrying, inefficiency of thinking, distractibility, anxiety, delusions, etc. The rating should be made on the basis of whether the symptom is present, not on what its cause is.

21. NEGLECT DUE TO BROODING

The subject is so preoccupied with unpleasant worries, fears or experiences, which are beyond his ability to stop, that he cannot cope with the affairs he should be dealing with. The effects are seen in quality and speed of work, whether domestic or vocational.

Moderate impairment includes a falling off in standard or speed of work. Severe impairment occurs when the subject has to take time off, or when a housewife is unable to complete some important part of her duties at all (such as shopping or cooking or cleaning or going to work).

22. RECENT LOSS OF INTEREST

There is a definite recent diminution in the subject's interests, either some interests have been dropped, or the intensity of interest has decreased. Everyone has interests of some sort but the extent of the diminution must be measured in the context of the range and depth of the subject's usual activities. Take into account everyday vocational and domestic activities as well as leisure pursuits, keeping well-informed, taking an interest in clothes, food and appearance, keeping up to date with the news, etc. Inevitably, those with the most intense and varied interests initially will have most room to lose interest and those who have never taken a great interest in things will not have much to lose.

'Recent loss' means 'within the present episode of illness'. If the subject began to be depressed two years ago, and his loss of interest dates from that time and is still present, include it. The rating of severity is still based on the past month. The extent of loss during the past month is compared with the usual level of interests two years ago.

23. DEPRESSED MOOD

Depressed mood may be expressed in a number of ways – sadness, misery, low spirits, inability to enjoy anything, dejection. (It may sometimes be expressed as apathy but this should be excluded from the present symptom unless the examiner is very sure of his ground. Depressive apathy may be included in the rating of 'depression on examination' – symptom no. 121.) The extent to which the subject has cried during the past month is one criterion of severity although it is not sufficient in itself (the deepest depression may be a frozen misery which is beyond tears). Another criterion of severity is lack of variability; moderate forms of depression tend to come and go more than severe forms.

Other forms of unpleasant affect (e.g. nervous tension, or anxiety) should be rated separately (e.g. symptoms 10 and 11). Depression may, of course, be present at the same time.

Criteria for rating (1)

Variable intensity; depression sometimes not very severe or even absent. May sometimes be deep depression but for brief periods of a few hours only. Occasional episodes of crying, often because of some upsetting incident. Cannot switch attention voluntarily to non-depressing topics, but attention can be directed to pleasanter topics (for example, by working hard, by the conversation of others, by chance happenings of an interesting kind).

Criteria for rating (2)

Deep depression lasts for long periods of time without variation. Episodes of crying for no reason at all. Mind almost totally occupied by depressing topics; very difficult to give attention to anything else, e.g. cannot be distracted by working harder, watching something interesting on the television, other people's conversation, etc.

24. HOPELESSNESS

The subject's view of the future is bleak and without comfort. Two degrees of intensity are distinguished by whether the patient has subjectively given up attempting to cope, because he can see no point in trying since the future is hopeless. A subject may say he feels hopeless but, at the same time, indicate that he continues to behave as though his life did contain some hope (moderate intensity – rate (1)). On the other hand, a subject may neglect himself and his affairs because of hopelessness (rate (2)) and, in the most severe case, attempt suicide.

Note that hopelessness is not always accompanied by depression.

25. SUICIDAL PLANS OR ACTS

This is one of the few items in the schedule with three degrees of severity. A fleeting thought about suicide is quite common and should not be rated. A more deliberate consideration of planning of possible techniques is rated (1). If a suicidal act is actually made, but there is some doubt as to whether it was really intended to result in the subject's death, rate (2). A serious attempt that the subject intended to result in death is rated (3).

26. ANXIETY OR DEPRESSION PRIMARY

If the subject suffers from both anxiety and depression, and both have been rated as being present, try to decide which is primary. The subject himself is quite often clear about the answer.

Anxiety is primary when any depression appears to be mainly explicable in terms of the limitations placed on the subject by his anxiety symptoms. Thus being unable to leave home or travel or meet people, or being afraid that palpitations mean heart disease, may be very depressing. The subject may be clear, however, that if the anxiety symptoms were not present the depression would vanish also. On the other hand the anxiety might well remain even if the depression disappeared. This situation is rated (0).

At the other extreme, the symptoms of anxiety may be reactive to the depressive condition – particularly if anxiety takes the form of fears of catastrophe, forebodings about illness or death, early morning dread at having to face the day, or a feeling that something awful is going to happen. Even when there are autonomic accompaniments, these anxiety symptoms may be seen quite clearly as secondary to depression – they would disappear if the depression did, but the depression would not necessarily be better if the anxiety disappeared. Anxiety due to fear of morbid or suicidal ideas is even more clearly secondary to depression. These conditions are rated (2).

In between these two fairly straightforward conditions, there are situations in which both anxiety and depression are present, but either they seem independent of each other or it is not possible to decide which one is primary. Rate these as (1).

27. MORNING DEPRESSION

The subject states unequivocally that depression is worst during the early part of the day and then improves. Characteristically, the subject wakes early and then lies awake feeling that he cannot get up and face the day. He has no appetite and crawls through the morning at a low tempo. Rate this condition (2).

If depression is not particularly marked in mornings, rate (1), and if no depression is present rate (0).

28. SOCIAL WITHDRAWAL

In the less intense form of the symptom, the subject does not seek company but does not refuse it when offered. In the more intense form, the subject actively withdraws and refuses company even when it is offered. Rate severity on a combination of intensity and frequency, consider only the past month, irrespective of how long the symptom has lasted.

29. SELF DEPRECIATION

The subject feels inferior to others, even – in the most intensive form of the symptom – worthless. Do not rate delusions here. Ideas of self-depreciation are an exaggerated form of self-knowledge about part of the subject's own character, which gives a false picture because not balanced by recognition that most human beings have similar faults. Self-depreciation implies a raising of the standard applied to the subject without an equivalent raising of the standard applied to others, or taking into account balancing merits.

Rate severity on a combination of intensity and frequency. Consider only the past month irrespective of how long the symptom has lasted.

30. LACK OF SELF-CONFIDENCE WITH PEOPLE

The subject lacks confidence in his social skills (do not take into account his confidence in mechanical or intellectual abilities). He anticipates discomfort and failure in matters which depend upon confidence in social relationships and feels that he is easily put upon by others. He does not feel himself to be a strong personality.

Rate severity in terms of frequency and intensity of symptom during the past month. Consider only the past month irrespective of how long the symptom has lasted. The symptom may well co-exist with no. 16 (autonomic anxiety on meeting people). If so, rate both.

31. SIMPLE IDEAS OF REFERENCE

In its moderate form, this symptom is indicated by selfconsciousness. The subject cannot help feeling that people take notice of him – in buses, in a restaurant, or in other public places – and that they observe things about him that he would prefer not to be seen. He realises that this feeling originates within himself and that he is no more noticed than other people, but cannot help the feeling all the same, quite out of proportion to any possible cause. This condition is rated (1), irrespective of how frequently it occurred during the month.

In its severe form, the subject thinks that people are critical of him, or that they tend to laugh at him. Often he is ashamed of something and cannot help feeling that others are aware of what it is. He realises that this feeling originates within himself. This condition is rated (2).

If the subject does, in fact, have some distinguishing physical characteristic which might cause him to be noticed rate (9) unless the subject's self-reference is out of all proportion.

Do not include delusions of reference (symptom no. 72) in which the subject believes that all sorts of events refer to him personally and has no insight into the origin of the self-reference within himself.

32. GUILTY IDEAS OF REFERENCE

The characteristics of 'simple ideas of reference' (symptom no. 31) are present but, in addition, the subject feels that he is blamed for some action or attribute. He realises that this feeling originates within himself but cannot help feeling it all the same, quite out of proportion to any possible cause. Rate this condition as (1) irrespective of frequency during the past month.

In the more intense form of the symptom, the subject actually feels that he is accused of some blameworthy action or attribute. He realises that this feeling originates within himself but cannot help feeling it all the same. Rate this condition as (2) irrespective of frequency during the past month.

If the subject has actually committed some blameworthy act which people are aware of, rate (9).

Do not include delusions of guilt (symptom no. 88) in which the subject thinks he deserves punishment for some crime that he has committed. Do not include pathological guilt, not amounting to delusions, which is not projected as an idea of reference (see symptom no. 33).

33. PATHOLOGICAL GUILT

The subject blames himself too much for some peccadillo which most people would not take very seriously. He realises that his guilt is exaggerated but cannot help feeling it all the same. Rate this condition (1) irrespective of frequency during the month. Do not include justifiable and appropriate guilt over some action which most people would agree was blameworthy. The guilt must be unpleasant, beyond voluntary control and out of proportion to the situation.

In the more intense form of the symptom the subject generalises the feeling of self-blame to almost anything that goes wrong in his environment. He realises that this guilt is exaggerated but cannot help feeling it all the same. Rate this condition (2) irrespective of frequency during the month.

Do not include delusions of guilt (symptom no. 88), in which the subject feels he has committed some terrible crime or is to blame for all the sins of the world, and has no insight into the origins of the symptom within his own mind.

34. LOSS OF WEIGHT

Rate only loss of weight due to poor appetite. If there is any organic illness which could account for it, rate (9). Consider weight loss during past three months only. Less than 15 kg (7 lbs) of loss is rated (1); 15 kg or more is rated (2).

35. DELAYED SLEEP

Rate delay in getting off to sleep after the subject has gone to bed. Rate one hour's delay as (1) and two hours delay as (2), irrespective of whether the patient is taking sleeping tablets. (Such medication should be noted on the front page of the schedule.) In either case, the sleeplessness must be fairly frequent, during the past month, say on ten or more nights (unless fewer were more or less consecutive, i.e. constituting an episode).

This symptom can co-exist with 'early waking' (symptom no. 37).

36. SUBJECTIVE ANERGIA AND RETARDATION

The subject feels that he has been slowed down in movement and/or has been markedly lacking in energy, compared to his usual condition. The symptom may have lasted since the onset of the episode of illness but it is rated only on the past month. Do not take into account the subject's speed of movement and response on examination (no. 110) – the symptom can only be rated on the subject's subjective account of how he feels.

Rate listlessness and lack of energy as (1), and marked feeling of retardation of movement and underactivity as (2), irrespective of frequency during the month.

37. EARLY WAKING

Rate waking one hour before usual time as (1) and two hours before usual time as (2), irrespective of whether subject is taking sleeping tablets (record this on front sheet of schedule). In either case, the early waking must be fairly frequent during the month, say on ten or more occasions (unless fewer were fairly consecutive: i.e. constituting an episode).

This symptom can co-exist with 'delayed sleep' (symptom no. 35).

38. LOSS OF LIBIDO

Compare with subject's normal level (which may be before onset of present episode of illness and therefore sometime ago) but rate only on the basis of past month. Thus if level of libido has been lower during past month than usual before onset of illness, rate 'loss' as (1) or (2) depending on lack of interest in sex, diminished frequency of intercourse, etc.

If any physical condition which might account for recent loss of libido, rate (9).

39. PREMENSTRUAL EXACERBATION

If subject is depressed or tense and complains that there is a definite exacerbation of these symptoms just before and at the start of menstruation, rate (1).

40. IRRITABILITY

Rate an increase in irritability during past month, compared with subject's norm (which may be before onset of present episode of illness some time ago). If this is mainly subjective and not externalised, rate (1). If it is shown by shouting or quarrelling, but without violence, rate (2). If it is shown by violent or destructive behaviour, rate (3). Rate according to the subject's own account, but remind the subject of anything written in the case-notes relating to his behaviour during past month. Do *not* rate positively if subject denies irritability (even if this is contradicted by case-notes).

41. EXPANSIVE MOOD

The subject is euphoric or elated for hours at a time, out of proportion to the circumstances he is in. *Do not include transient high spirits concordant with circumstances.* There is usually an element of excitement or of irritability which the patient may recognise as disturbing or unhealthy. Occasionally the symptom may be more transient but very frequently repeated – it may then still be rated as present.

An element of judgement is required for this rating since the subject often does not recognise his mood as having been expansive once the mood is past, but may simply describe himself as having been cheerful or in ordinary good spirits. Do not set the threshold of the symptom too low, but take into account the context of other symptoms and any note about mood in the case-record.

This is one of the symptoms of the PSE where clinical judgement is particularly important. If the symptom seems likely to have been present during the month, even though not explicitly described by the subject rate (1). If the patient does describe the symptom, rate (2) irrespective of frequency.

42. SUBJECTIVE IDEOMOTOR PRESSURE

This symptom is the subjective aspect of flight of ideas. Images and ideas flash through the mind, each suggesting others, at a fast rate. The state persists for hours or longer at a time. If the subject describes any episode of this kind, rate (1) irrespective of frequency during the past month.

A more intense form of the symptom is when it becomes expressed in motor behaviour. The subject has tremendous energy, is far more active than usual, his movements are rapid and he does not need so much sleep as usual. Rate (2) in this case, irrespective of frequency during the past month.

43. GRANDIOSE IDEAS AND ACTIONS

The subject feels that he is superbly healthy, has exceptionally high intelligence or extraordinary abilities. If this has occurred during the past month, rate (1) irrespective of frequency. If the ideas have been translated into action, e.g. overspending, gambling, etc., rate (2) irrespective of frequency. Remind the subject, if necessary, of items recorded in case-notes.

Do not include 'compulsive gambling' unless clearly based on expansive mood and grandiose ideas.

The borderline between this symptom and 'grandiose delusions' (symptoms nos. 76 and 77) is difficult to draw except that grandiose ideas are simply exaggerations of the subject's normal state (e.g. he may actually be capable and intelligent or have some particular ability) whereas delusions involve an identification or an assertion that is demonstrably false (e.g. that he is a king or that he invented the atom-bomb). In either case, however, insight tends to be lacking.

44. OBSESSIONAL CHECKING AND REPEATING

The central feature of an obsessional symptom must be present, that is that the checking or repetitive action is experienced as being carried out against conscious resistance. He is impelled to check light switches or gas taps many times (not just two or three times), to touch or count things or to repeat the same action over and over again.

Rate according to intensity and frequency during the past month.

After a very long time the experience of conscious resistance may begin to lose its force if the subject habitually yields to the impulse – but the nature of the symptom is by then quite obvious.

45. OBSESSIONAL CLEANLINESS AND RITUALS

The central feature of an obsessional symptom must be present, that is that the fear of contamination, or the handwashing or other ritual, is experienced as being carried out against conscious resistance. The subject recognises that it is senseless and tries to resist it but cannot. He is compelled to wash, or to avoid touching things in case of contamination, or to carry out other complex rituals to do with cleanliness, over and over again.

Rate according to intensity and frequency during the past month.

After a very long time the experience of conscious resistance may begin to lose its force if the subject habitually yields to the impulse – but the nature of the symptom is by then quite obvious.

46. OBSESSIONAL IDEAS AND RUMINATION

The central feature of an obsessional symptom must be present, that is the ideas enter the mind against conscious resistance. The subject tries to resist it but cannot.

He is impelled to think of certain ideas or images (e.g. knives or obscenities) or to ruminate constantly upon the meaning of the universe.

Rate according to intensity and frequency during the past month.

After a very long time the experience of conscious resistance may begin to lose its force if the subject habitually yields to the impulse but the nature of the symptom is by then quite obvious.

47. DEREALISATION

The subject experiences his surroundings as unreal. An office or a bus or a street seem like a stage set with actors, rather than real people going about their ordinary business. Everything seems colourless, artificial and dead.

In the less intense form of the symptom, the subject simply experiences a lack of colour and life, so that any tendency towards the artificial tends to be exaggerated. People seem to be pretending their emotions. Rate this condition as (1) irrespective of frequency during the month. In a more severe form of the symptom, the subject feels 'as though the world is made of plastic', 'as though it is not really there at all', as though 'people are puppets on strings without any real life of their own'. Rate this condition as (2) irrespective of frequency during the month.

The subject retains a measure of understanding and knows the condition is abnormal.

Do not include any delusional explanation or elaboration of this experience in the rating.

48. DEPERSONALISATION

Derealisation (symptom no. 47) is often present at the same time and should be rated independently. The subject feels as if he himself is unreal, that he is acting a part rather than being spontaneous and natural, that he is a sham, a shadow of a real person. He feels detached from his experiences, as though he were viewing them from a long way off, or through the wrong end of a telescope. This condition should be rated (1), irrespective of frequency during the month.

A more severe form of the symptom occurs when the subject feels as if he were actually dead. He may feel that when he looks in the mirror he cannot see a proper reflection, or that part of his body does not belong to him, or that he is living in some entirely different 'parallel world' and cannot interact in this one. Rate this condition as (2), irrespective of frequency during the month.

The subject retains a measure of understanding and knows the condition is abnormal. Do not include delusional explanation or elaboration of this experience in the rating (see symptom no. 90, when symptom has delusional force).

49. DELUSIONAL MOOD

The subject feels that his familiar surroundings have changed in a puzzling way, which he may be unable to describe, but which seems to be specially significant for him. He may simply say that everything seems odd and strange and that he can't understand what is going on. He may experience this as ominous or threatening or simply appear puzzled. This condition is rated as (1) irrespective of frequency during the past month. If the subject attempts an explanation, it is likely to be either that he is becoming ill, still rated as (1), or to be couched in the form of delusions, rated (2). Often the meaning of these puzzling feelings becomes clear to the subject when a delusional concept or a delusion is formed. Rate (2) only when this crystal-lisation has occurred during the past month. Differentiate from derealisation and depersonalisation.

50. HEIGHTENED PERCEPTION

Sounds seem unnaturally clear or loud or intense, colours appear more brilliant or beautiful, details of the environment seem to stand out in a particularly interesting way, and any sensation may be experienced exceptionally vividly. The pattern on a wallpaper, or the cracks in a ceiling, may become insistently noticeable. Once the experience is past, the subject often finds it difficult to remember or describe, and the examiner must use judgement to rate its presence. In such a case, rate (1). If it has quite clearly and definitely been present during the past month, even briefly, rate (2). The symptom should be rated present only when there is a definite per-ceptual change, e.g. lack of interest would not qualify.

51. DULLED PERCEPTION

This symptom is the opposite of 'heightened perception' (symptom no. 50). The subject experiences things as dark or grey, uniform and uninteresting and flat. Tastes and appetites are blunted, colours may appear to be muddy or dirty, sounds to be ugly or impure. Once the symptom has disappeared it may be difficult for the subject to remember or describe it and the examiner must use judgement to rate its presence – in such a case, rate (1). If the symptom has quite clearly and definitely been present during the past month, even if briefly, rate (2).

52. CHANGED PERCEPTION

Include here any change in perception that is not included under symptoms 50 and 51 ('heightened and dulled perception'). The subject may complain that objects change in shape or size or colour or that people change their appearance. Once the symptom has disappeared it may be difficult for the subject to remember or describe it and the examiner must use judgement to rate its presence – in such a case, rate (1). If the symptom has quite clearly and definitely been present during the past month, even if briefly, rate (2).

53. CHANGED PERCEPTION OF TIME

The subject's perception of time seems to change, so that events appear to move very slowly or very rapidly or to change their tempo or to be completely timeless.

Include the experience that events appear to happen exactly as they happened before, so that the subject feels that he has relived them exactly (deja vu). Time may appear to stop altogether. Once the symptom has disappeared it may be difficult for the subject to remember or describe it and the examiner must use judgement to rate its presence – in such a case, rate (1). If the symptom has quite clearly and definitely been present during the past month, even if briefly, rate (2).

54. LOSS OF AFFECT

The subject complains that he has lost the ability to feel, to experience emotion. He can remember a time when he did have this capacity (though it might have been months or years ago) and is quite clear about losing it. Rate only if the symptom has been present during the past month. Rate severity on the basis of intensity and frequency during the past month. The symptom may be associated with depression (particularly chronic depressive apathy) and other affects. It is a subjective complaint and should not be confused with blunting of affect (symptom no. 128).

55. THOUGHT INSERTION

This symptom is frequently recorded as present on inadequate evidence. Subjects often answer affirmatively to the initial question without having understood it. If examiners too, do not have the specific symptom in mind but some more general approximation to it, and thus fail to ask the most important extra questions, there are bound to be errors in rating. The symptom is very significant diagnostically and so the greatest care must be taken never to rate it as present without good evidence and a written example.

The essence of the symptom is that the subject experiences thoughts *which are not his own* intruding into his mind. The symptom is not that he has been caused to have unusual thoughts (for example, if he thinks the Devil is making him think evil thoughts) but that the thoughts *themselves* are not his. In the most typical case, the alien thoughts are said to have been inserted into the mind from outside, by means of radar or telepathy or some other means: rate this (2). In such a case there is an explanatory delusion as well (symptoms no. 78–81). However, a rating of (2) does not depend upon the presence of an explanatory delusion, but simply on the conviction that alien thoughts are present which have been inserted from outside.

Sometimes the subject may say that he does not know where the alien thoughts came from, although he is quite clear that they are not his own. In very rare instances, he may postulate that they come from his own unconscious mind – while still consciously experiencing them as alien. Rate these situations (1).

Several confusing problems, often leading to a false positive rating, are discussed below:

(i)   Some subjects, because of an inadequate intellectual level or poor verbal ability, are quite unable to grasp what is being asked, or to give a rateable answer. In such cases, do *not* give the benefit of the doubt: make full use of (8), if there is some possibility that the symptom has not been excluded or (9), if it is quite impossible to tell.

(ii) Neurotic symptoms such as 'inefficient thinking' (no. 19), 'ideomotor pressure' (no. 24) and 'brooding' (no. 21) are often confused by patients for the symptom. The examiner should have no difficulty, however, since in none of these cases are alien thoughts experienced as being inserted into the mind.

(iii) Auditory pseudohallucinations (voices experienced as being within the mind) may be very difficult to distinguish since sometimes the subject is unable to say whether the experience is a voice or a thought. In such cases rate both symptoms as present. (If the experience is of a voiced thought not alien to the subject, rate on symptom no. 56.)

(iv) The subject may explain the experience of thought insertion in delusional terms (e.g. due to hypnotism or telepathy). In such a case rate both symptoms as present. However, if the subject merely complains that he is being influenced, or even simply that his thoughts are being read, take care! A delusion of influence is *not* the same as thought insertion. In particular, a delusion that a subject's thoughts are being read or that telepathy or hypnotism is going on (no. 59), often does *not* mean that he experiences thoughts being inserted. He often means that somehow people seem to know what he is thinking (either they can infer his thoughts from his behaviour, or they seem to have extraordinary powers). Similarly, delusions of religious influence do not mean thought insertion *ipso facto*: although the content of his thinking is influenced by God or the Devil, etc., his thoughts are his own thoughts.

(v) An elated subject may speak as if his thoughts were coming from elsewhere – e.g. they are so magnificent that it seems as if they must have come from the sun, so good that they must have come from God, etc. But in such cases the subject knows they are his thoughts. If he describes them as 'God's' thoughts, this is only a manner of speaking.

56. THOUGHT BROADCAST OR THOUGHT SHARING

See definition of 'thought insertion' (no. 55): the general remarks apply also to the present symptom which is often rated positively on insufficient evidence.

Rate (1) if the subject says that his own thoughts seem to sound 'aloud' in his head, almost as though someone standing nearby could hear them ('gedankenlaut-werden'). If thoughts are *repeated*, rate as symptom no. 57.

Rate (2) if the subject experiences his thoughts actually being shared with others, often with large numbers of people (irrespective of the mechanism; but this is usually said to be some form of 'broadcasting').

The symptom is a rare one. Distinguish it from thought reading. Subjects quite often say their thoughts are being read, without having had the experience of thought broadcast. What they mean is that other people can tell from their expression, or from their habits, what they are likely to be thinking. Thought reading can also be an explanatory delusion. For example, if the subject has an extensive system of delusions of reference so that wherever he goes he seems to be followed, or people are making signs at him, he may say that whoever is organising it can read his thoughts, thus knowing where he is going to go and how to instruct others to react to him. 'Thought broadcast' is only rated when the subject actually experiences his thoughts being shared with others. There is very rarely any doubt when the symptom is present – even a rather unintelligent or uneducated patient can describe it quite accurately.

Distinguish from pseudohallucinations (no. 65) in which the subject hears voices within his mind, not through the ears. The voice is not, however, said to be the subject's own thoughts.

Distinguish also from thought withdrawal (no. 58) in which thoughts are not experienced as broadcast or shared, but as withdrawn so that the subject has no thoughts.

57. THOUGHT ECHO OR COMMENTARY

See definition of 'thought insertion' (no. 55): the general remarks apply also to the present symptom which is often rated positively on insufficient evidence.

The subject experiences his own thought as repeated or echoed (not just spoken aloud = 56) with very little interval between the original and the echo. Rate this situation (1). The repetition may not be a simple echo, however, but subtly or grossly changed in quality.

If the subject experiences alien thoughts in association with his own, or as comments upon his own, rate (2). This experience is very rare but, when it occurs, the subject can describe it exactly. It is not the same as voices commenting on the subject's thoughts (no. 64).

58. THOUGHT BLOCK OR THOUGHT WITHDRAWAL

Thought block is extremely rare and should only be rated present when the examiner is quite sure it is present. If there is any doubt, it is probably *not* present. The subject experiences a sudden stopping of his thoughts, quite unexpectedly, while they are flowing freely, and in the absence of anxiety. When it occurs it is fairly dramatic and it happens on several occasions. Rate this (1).

Although the subject may be unable to describe pure thought block, it is very recognisable in the form of an explanatory delusion of thought withdrawal. The subject says that his thoughts have been removed from his head so that he has no thoughts.

Distinguish from the somewhat similar delusion of depersonalisation (no. 90) in which the subject may say that he has no thought, but not that his thoughts have suddenly stopped or that they have withdrawn. It is the element of withdrawal which makes the symptom recognisable – rate (2). Withdrawal may be present without thought block being experienced.

Distinguish also from thought broadcast or sharing (no. 56) in which the subject still has plenty of thoughts but experiences them as being available to others besides himself.

59. DELUSIONS OF THOUGHT BEING READ

This is usually an explanatory delusion. Often it goes with delusions of reference or misinterpretation, which require some explanation of how other people know so much about the subject's future movements. It may be an elaboration of thought broadcast, thought insertion, auditory hallucinations, delusions of control, delusions of persecution or delusions of influence. It can even occur with expansive delusions (the subject wishing to explain how Einstein, for example, stole his original ideas). The symptom is therefore in no way diagnostic. It is most important that it should not be mistaken for diagnostically more important symptoms such as thought insertion or broadcast.

If the subject merely entertains the possibility that his thought might be read but is not certain about it, rate (1). Rate delusional conviction (2).

Exclude those who think that people can read their thoughts as a result of belonging to a group that practices 'thought reading' – this would be rated (1) or (2) on symptom no. 83.

60. NON-VERBAL HALLUCINATIONS

This symptom includes noises, other than words, which have no real origin in the world outside the subject but also no explicable origin in bodily processes, and which the subject regards as separate from his own mental processes. Thus tinnitus or the sound of the subject's heart beating are not included, nor is the memory of a piece of music. Consciousness is clear. Any auditory hallucinations taking the form of recognisable words are excluded.

Rate (1) if the subject hears noises such as music, tapping, central heating noises, etc., when they demonstrably are not occurring in reality and are not part of the subject's memories or voluntary imaginings. Rate (2) if the subject hears whispering, muttering or mumbling but cannot make out the words (though occasionally he may 'know' what is being said without hearing the words). If there are recognisable words as well – rate one or more of the other symptoms concerning auditory hallucinations (nos. 61, 62, 63, 64), whichever are applicable. Include both true and pseudohallucinations.

61. AFFECTIVE OR NON-SPECIFIC VERBAL HALLUCINATIONS

This symptom excludes non-verbal auditory hallucinations (symptom no. 60). The most common form of the symptom is a voice calling the subject's name or simply saying one or two words only (often someone with whom the subject has or had strong affective ties; the typical situation is shortly after a bereavement). Consciousness is clear. Rate this condition (1). If the subject hears a voice, or voices, speaking directly to him, with content which is purely depressive (e.g. depreciatory, and often thought to be deserved), rate (2). If the content is congruent with an elated mood (e.g. 'Go to the palace, they will make you king'), rate (3). Include both true and pseudohallucinations. Rate (1) if the subject entertains the possibility of a voice but is not certain, or thinks that it might be due to his own unconscious mental processes. Always write down an example.

Be careful to distinguish this symptom from delusions of reference (no. 72) in which the subject thinks that other people talk about him, usually disparagingly, because he thinks he sees them glance meaningfully at him while talking amongst themselves, or thinks that some remark is dropped which is meant especially for him, but does not actually hear the words spoken. In most such cases, the subject is not experiencing auditory hallucinations but making a delusional misinterpretation. If in doubt in such a situation, do not rate both auditory hallucinations and delusions of reference as present but use (8). Illusions, as when a subject thinks he hears his name called in a crowd, should be excluded.

62. NON-AFFECTIVE VERBAL HALLUCINATIONS (ABOUT THE SUBJECT)

This symptom includes only a voice or voices heard by the subject speaking about him and therefore referring to him in the third person. Consciousness is clear. The content is not depressive or grandiose in keeping with the mood. (Exclude for example, 'This man is evil, we must hang him'.) Include both true and pseudohallucinations. Rate (8) if the example given by the subject contains only one or two sentences since it is usually impossible to judge with any certainty whether the basis is affective or subcultural or not.

Rate (1) if the subject hears the voice commenting on his thoughts or actions, and thus speaking about him in the third person. Rate (2) if the subject hears voices talking to each other about him in the third person. Always write down an example.

Be careful to distinguish the symptom from delusions of reference (no. 72), in which the subject thinks that other people talk about him, usually disparagingly, because he thinks he sees them glance meaningfully at him while talking amongst themselves, or thinks that some remark is dropped which is meant especially for him, but does not actually hear the words spoken. In most such cases, the subject is not experiencing auditory hallucinations but making a delusional misinterpretation. If in doubt in such a situation, do not rate both auditory hallucinations and delusions of reference, but give preference to the latter.

63. NON-AFFECTIVE VERBAL HALLUCINATIONS (SPOKEN TO THE SUBJECT)

This symptom includes only a voice or voices heard by the subject speaking directly to him, and not depressive or grandiose in content and mood. Consciousness is clear. Include both true and pseudohallucinations. Rate (1) if the tone and content are pleasant, supportive or neutral but not based upon affective change. Rate (2) if the tone and content are hostile or threatening or accusatory but not based upon affective change. Always write down an example.

Do not include voices saying one or two words only, or the content of whose remarks is depressive or grandiose in keeping with the subject's mood (symptom no. 61).

Do not include voices which talk about the subject in the third person (symptom no. 63).

Be careful to distinguish the symptom from delusions of reference (no. 72), in which the subject thinks that other people talk about him, usually disparagingly, because he thinks he sees them glance meaningfully at him while talking amongst themselves, or thinks that some remark is dropped which is meant especially for him, but does not actually hear the words spoken. In most such cases, the subject is not experiencing auditory hallucinations but making a delusional misinterpretation. If in doubt in such a situation, do not rate both auditory hallucinations and delusions of reference, but give preference to the latter.

64. 'DISSOCIATIVE' HALLUCINATIONS

The subject can hold a conversation (often two-way) with a presence (variously described as a person, ghost, spirit, god, etc.) which may often be sensed in other ways, e.g. visually or by touch or smell. Often connected with people with whom the subject has had strong affective ties. Visual hallucinations can occur alone. There is either a strong subcultural colouring, e.g. the subject belongs to a religious sect or to a subcultural group which sanctions hallucinatory experiences, or the subject has been under the influence of someone who is involved with such practices. Exclude hypnogogic hallucinations.

Rate (1) if 'dissociative' hallucinations are present and the subject belongs to a subcultural group or sect in which such experiences are sanctioned. Rate (2) if 'dissociative' hallucinations are present but the subject does not belong to such a subcultural group. Usually, in such a case, there will be a history of contact with some individual who has been involved with such experiences, or possibly with a book, film, etc., which deals with them.

If there is any doubt about the nature of the hallucinations, use (8). Do not rate symptoms (61), (62), (63) or (66) as present, if the experiences fall within the present category. See note on possession states in the definition of symptom 71.

65. TRUE OR PSEUDOHALLUCINATIONS

The distinction between true and pseudohallucinations depends upon whether the subject hears the voice(s) within his mind or outside it. True hallucinations are experienced as coming from outside the mind and are heard through the ears. Pseudohallucinations are heard within the mind, not coming from the outside and not experienced in objective space.

This symptom should be rated in all cases in which the patient is rated as having auditory hallucinations (symptoms nos. 61, 62, 63 and 64).

66. VISUAL HALLUCINATIONS (CLEAR CONSCIOUSNESS)

The subject sees objects, people, images which other people cannot see. Consciousness is clear. The vision may appear to be in the external world (true hallucination) or within the subject's own mind (pseudohallucination). Rate this condition (2). If the subject simply sees formless images, shadows, coloured lights, rate (1). Always write down an example. Distinguish however from misinterpretations of real stimuli (such as an anxious person thinking there is an intruder in the shadows). The visual equivalent of symptom 61 (e.g. a subject who sees her recently dead husband) should not be rated here. Make a separate note.

67. VISUAL HALLUCINATIONS (CLOUDED CONSCIOUSNESS)

Consciousness is clouded. The subject may have almost any variety of visual experience from complete scenes witnessed as on a stage to flashes of light. Small animals are not particularly characteristic. Rate unformed hallucinations – flashes of light, coloured zig zags or stars, etc. as (1). Rate formed hallucinations as (2). Include both true and pseudohallucinations. Always write down an example.

68. OLFACTORY HALLUCINATIONS AND DELUSIONS

Simple olfactory hallucinations, such as a smell of orange peel or perfume, or a smell of 'death' or burning, which other people cannot smell, are rated (1). Be sure that there is no more obvious cause (sinusitis, or a misinterpretation of a smell that really is present). If the experience is delusionally elaborated, e.g. the subject not only smells gas but thinks that gas is deliberately being let into the room, rate (2). Always write down an example.

If the subject thinks that he himself smells, rate symptom no. 69. The symptoms can of course co-exist.

69. DELUSION THAT SUBJECT SMELLS

If the subject thinks that he gives off a smell (though others cannot smell it) but is uncertain, or simply thinks it possible, rate (1). Exclude preoccupation with body odour, e.g. in an anxious subject who sweats a lot. If the subject is certain that he gives off a smell and that others notice it and react accordingly, rate (2).

Distinguish from other olfactory hallucinations and delusional elaborations (symptom no. 68).

70. OTHER HALLUCINATIONS AND DELUSIONAL ELABORATIONS

If the subject has sensations other than auditory, visual, sexual or olfactory – e.g. food tastes burnt or acid, something seems to touch him, ants seem to crawl over his skin – but does not delusionally elaborate, rate (1). Exclude other obvious explanations for the experience. If the subject elaborates in a delusional way (e.g. food poisoned, etc.) – rate (2). Always write down an example. The equivalent of symptom 61 (e.g. a subject who senses her dead husband to be momentarily present and feels him touch her) should not be rated here. Make a separate note. Sexual hallucinations should be rated as symptom 86.

PARTIAL AND FULL DELUSIONS

Most delusional symptoms are rated according to whether there is partial or full conviction. Partial delusions are expressed with doubt, as a possibility which the subject is prepared to entertain but is not certain about. If the subject has had full conviction during the past month, e.g. if he has acted as though the delusional belief were true, the rating should be (2) irrespective of the degree of conviction at the time of interview. However, if the delusion does not seem to have been formed fully but is still at the stage of being only one conceivable explanation for some unusual experience, rate (1).

71. DELUSIONS OF CONTROL

This is a symptom (like thought insertion and thought broadcast) which tends to be rated present when it is in fact absent. The essence of the symptom is that the subject experiences his will as replaced by that of some other force or agency. Unless the examiner is confident that the subject has indeed had this experience during the past month, the symptom is absent. When in doubt, rate (8), (9), or (0), according to circumstances, *not* (1).

The basic experience may be elaborated in various ways – the subject believes that someone else's words are coming out using his voice, or that what he writes is not his own, or that he is the victim of possession – a zombie or a robot controlled by someone else's will, even his bodily movements being willed by some other power. A partial delusion is rated (1) and a full delusion (2). Partial delusions are expressed with doubt, as a possibility which the subject is prepared to entertain but is not certain about. If the subject has had full conviction during the past month, e.g. if he has acted as though the delusional belief were true, the rating should be (2) irrespective of the degree of conviction at the time of interview. However, if the delusion does not seem to have formed fully but is still at the stage of being only one conceivable explanation for some unusual experience, rate (1). Always write down an example.

A simple statement that the subject is 'being controlled' or 'being influenced' is not sufficient to rate the symptom as present. The subject may mean only that his life is planned and directed by fate or that the future is already present in embryo or that he is not very strong-willed. He may mean that voices are giving him orders. He may mean that he thinks that God is omnipotent and controls everything, himself included, or that he himself is God (this is a religious delusion – symptom no. 78). None of these alternatives should be included if the essential element is missing. Only close cross-questioning can establish whether delusions of control are indeed present.

Do not include if an elated subject says he is 'under God's control' meaning that his will, far from being replaced, is greatly strengthened, *as if* it were God's.

If the subject describes a socially shared experience, or one which is explicable purely in subcultural terms, rate symptom no. 83. For example, a Taoist priestess who said that she was controlled by the God when she was in a trance would not be rated as having delusions of control.

NOTE ON 'POSSESSION' STATES (RELEVANT TO SYMPTOMS 64, 71, 83, 100, 102)

The difference between subcultural or hysterical possession states and delusions of control (symptom 71) lies first in the state of consciousness. The former occur in a state of dissociation which is rated as symptom 100 (or symptom 102 if it amounts to stupor). The latter occur in clear consciousness. A second differentiating point is that the subcultural possession state is a culturally normative experience, that is, the subject's claim to be possessed is endorsed by other members of his group. The hysterical possession state may not be so endorsed but its subcultural origins should still be clear and the motivation for the symptom will usually be obvious. A delusion of control should not be rated present if there is any doubt on these two points (use (8) if the issue is genuinely undecided, or (9) if it is impossible to make a judgement). A third point is that subcultural possession states are ego-enhancing in their effect, since the subject becomes identified with a more powerful being. Delusions of control, however, express an experience of loss rather than acquisition of identity and they are often based on other abnormal experiences, rated elsewhere.

Rate the dissociative state as symptom 100 or 102. Rate the experience of possession as symptom 83. Rate dissociative hallucinations as symptom 64. These can all be present together and are then all rated. However, they can also occur singly as, for example, in the attribution of physical illness or states of discomfort to influence by an evil spirit, without any trance phenomena.

72. DELUSIONS OF REFERENCE

Ideas of self-reference are rated in symptoms no. 31 and 32. Delusions of reference consist of a further elaboration of this experience in so far as other people are involved. Thus what is said may have a double meaning, or someone makes a gesture which the subject construes as a deliberate message, e.g. someone crossing his legs may be taken to mean that the subject is a homosexual. The whole neighbourhood may seem to be gossiping about the subject, far beyond the bounds of possibility, or he may see references to himself on the television or in newspapers. The subject may hear someone on the radio say something connected with some topic that he has just been thinking about (incidentally, this is *not* thought broadcast, which is a specific experience and should be rated separately as symptom no. 56). The subject may seem to be followed, his movements observed and what he says tape-recorded. Rate partial delusions as (1) and full delusional conviction as (2). Partial delusions are expressed with doubt, as a possibility which the subject is prepared to entertain but is not certain about. If the subject has had full conviction during the past month, e.g. if he has acted as though the delusional belief were true, the rating should be (2) irrespective of the degree of conviction at the time of interview. However, if the delusion does not seem to have formed fully but is still at the stage of being only one conceivable explanation for some unusual experience, rate (1). Delusions of reference may be based upon guilt (people are blaming or accusing the subject) or upon elation (they are interested in the subject because he is so important or noteworthy) or they may be primary delusions - sudden convictions that a particular gesture or set of events refer to the subject and have a special significance. Rate all these together in the one symptom, but rate primary delusions in addition under symptom no. 82. See the next symptom, delusions of misinterpretation, for an extension of this symptom to other situations.

See also auditory hallucinations (particularly symptoms no. 61–4). It is, of course, possible for a subject to have both symptoms but they are not identical. If the subject thinks people are talking about him, or making remarks intended for him to overhear, when they are in his presence, it is most likely that he is misinterpreting, not hearing voices. Careful questioning should enable the examiner to judge whether one or other or both symptoms are present.

73. DELUSIONAL MISINTERPRETATION AND MISIDENTIFICATION

This symptom is a further extension of the delusion of reference in that not only do people seem to refer to the subject directly but situations seem to be created which have a special meaning. Things seem to be arranged to test him out, objects are arranged so that they have a special significance for him, street signs or advertisements on buses or patterns of colour seem to have been put there in order to give him a message. This may go so far that whole armies of people may seem to be employed simply in order to discover what he is doing, or to convey some message to him. He may think he sees people he knew in the distant past, specially planted in his way so as to remind him of something. The subject does not necessarily feel persecuted or grandiose or interpret in some other delusional way. He may simply be puzzled as to why these events are going on. Rate (1) if partial delusions and (2) if full delusional conviction. Partial delusions are expressed with doubt, as a possibility which the subject is prepared to entertain but is not certain about. If the subject has had full conviction during the past month, e.g. if he has acted as though the delusional belief were true, the rating should be (2) irrespective of the degree of conviction at the time of interview. However, if the delusion does not seem to have formed fully but is still at the stage of being only one conceivable explanation for some unusual experience, rate (1). Always write down an example.

74. DELUSIONS OF PERSECUTION

The subject believes that someone, or some organisation, or some force or power, is trying to harm him in some way; to damage his reputation, to cause him bodily injury, to drive him mad or to bring about his death.

The symptom may take many forms from the direct belief that people are hunting him down to complex and bizarre plots with every kind of science fiction elaboration. Rate partial delusions as (1) and full delusional conviction as (2). Partial delusions are expressed with doubt, as a possibility which the subject is prepared to entertain but is not certain about. If the subject had had full conviction during the past month, e.g. if he has acted as though the delusional belief were true, the rating should be (2) irrespective of the degree of conviction at the time of the interview. However, if the delusion does not seem to have formed fully but is still at the stage of being only one conceivable explanation for some unusual experience, rate (1). Always write down an example.

A simple delusion of reference, e.g. that the subject is being followed or spied upon, is not included (see symptom no. 72) unless the subject believes that harm is intended, in which case rate both symptoms as present.

75. DELUSIONS OF ASSISTANCE

The subject believes that someone, or some organisation, or some force or power, is trying to help him. This delusion may arise as an explanation for the experiences which are expressed as delusions of reference (in the same way that delusions of persecution can arise). Delusions of assistance may be simple (people make signs to the subject in order to persuade him to be a better person, because they want to help him) or complicated (angels organise everything so that the subject's life is directed in the most advantageous way). Grandiose or religious delusions may be present at the same time. Rate partial delusions as (1) and full delusional conviction as (2). Partial delusions are expressed with doubt, as a possibility which the subject is prepared to entertain but is not certain about. If the subject has had full conviction during the past month, e.g. if he has acted as though the delusional belief were true, the rating should be (2) irrespective of the degree of conviction at the time of interview. However, if the delusion does not seem to have formed fully but is still at the stage of being only one conceivable explanation for some unusual experience, rate (1). Always write down an example.

76. DELUSIONS OF GRANDIOSE ABILITY

The subject thinks he is chosen by some power, or by destiny, for a special mission or purpose, because of his unusual talents. He thinks he is able to read people's thoughts, or that he is particularly good at helping them, that he is much cleverer than anyone else, that he has invented machines, composed music, solved mathematical problems, etc. beyond most people's comprehension. Partial delusions are rated (1) and full delusional conviction as (2). Partial delusions are expressed with doubt, as a possibility which the subject is prepared to entertain but is not certain about. If the subject has had full conviction during the past month, e.g. if he has acted as though the delusional belief were true, the rating should be (2) irrespective of the degree of conviction at the time of interview. However, if the delusion does not seem to have formed fully but is still at the stage of being only one conceivable explanation for some unusual experience, rate (1). Always write down an example.

77. DELUSIONS OF GRANDIOSE IDENTITY

The subject believes he is famous, rich, titled or related to prominent people. He may believe that he is a changeling and that his real parents are royalty, etc. Partial delusions are rated as (1) and full delusional conviction as (2). Partial delusions are expressed with doubt, as a possibility which the subject is prepared to entertain but is not certain about. If the subject has had full conviction during the past month e.g. if he has acted as though the delusional belief were true, the rating should be (2) irrespective of the degree of conviction at the time of interview. However, if the delusion does not seem to have formed fully but is still at the stage of being only one conceivable explanation for some unusual experience, rate (1). Always write down an example.

Do not include an identification with God or a saint or an angel as grandiose – this should be counted as a religious delusion (no. 78).

78. RELIGIOUS DELUSIONS

Both a religious identification on the part of a subject (he is a saint or has special spiritual powers) and an explanation in religious terms of other abnormal experiences (e.g. auditory hallucinations) should be included. Partial delusions are rated (1) and full delusional conviction is rated (2). Partial delusions are expressed with doubt, as a possibility which the subject is prepared to entertain but is not certain about. If the subject has had full conviction during the past month, e.g. if he has acted as though the delusional belief were true, the rating should be (2) irrespective of the degree of conviction at the time of interview. However, if the delusion does not seem to have formed fully but is still at the stage of being only conceivable explanation for some unusual experience, rate (1). Always write down an example.

Exclude an intense degree of ordinary religious conviction and exclude any special subcultural religious beliefs (e.g. 'speaking in tongues' if the subject belongs to a particular church). Rate the latter as symptom no. 83.

79. DELUSIONAL EXPLANATIONS (PARANORMAL AND OCCULT)

Include here any delusional explanation or elaboration of other abnormal experiences, such as thought insertion or broadcast or delusions of reference or persecution, in terms of paranormal phenomena. Include explanations in terms of hypnotism, telepathy, magic, witchcraft, etc. Rate partial delusions (1) and full delusional conviction (2). Partial delusions are expressed with doubt, as a possibility which the subject is prepared to entertain but is not certain about. If the subject has had full conviction during the past month, e.g. if he has acted as though the delusional belief were true, the rating should be (2) irrespective of the degree of conviction at the time of interview. However, if the delusion does not seem to have formed fully but is still at the stage of being only one conceivable explanation for some unusual experience, rate (1). Always write down an example.

Exclude ideas which are accepted by a sub-cultural group and derived solely from membership in that group – rate these as part of symptom 82.

80. DELUSIONAL EXPLANATIONS (PHYSICAL)

Include here any delusional explanation of other abnormal experiences such as thought insertion or broadcast or delusions of reference or persecution or somatic delusions, in terms of physical processes such as electricity, X-rays, television, radio or machines of various kind. Rate partial delusions (1) and full delusional conviction (2). Partial delusions are expressed with doubt, as a possibility which the subject is prepared to entertain but is not certain about. If the subject has had full conviction during the past month, e.g. if he has acted as though the delusional belief were true, the rating should be (2) irrespective of the degree of conviction at the time of interview. However, if the delusion does not seem to have formed fully but is still at the stage of being only one conceivable explanation for some unusual experience, rate (1). Always write down an example.

81. DELUSION OF ALIEN FORCES PENETRATING OR CONTROLLING MIND OR BODY

This symptom is rated on the basis of an experience which will already have been rated elsewhere. This involves an external force which penetrates the subject's mind or body from outside – such as a ray which turns the liver to gold, alien thoughts which pierce the skull or are injected into the mind, or a spirit which speaks with the subject's voice, or a radio transmitter which has been implanted into the brain so that the subject's thoughts are broadcast, etc. Rate partial delusions as (1) and full delusional conviction as (2). Partial delusions are expressed with doubt, as a possibility which the subject is prepared to entertain but is not certain about. If the subject has had full conviction during the past month, e.g. if he has acted as though the delusional belief were true, the rating should be (2) irrespective of the degree of conviction at the time of interview. However, if the delusion does not seem to have formed fully but is still at the stage of being only one conceivable explanation for some unusual experience, rate (1). Always write down an example.

82. PRIMARY DELUSIONS

Primary delusions are based upon sensory experiences (delusional perceptions) in which a patient suddenly becomes convinced that a particular set of events has a special meaning. For example, a subject undergoing liver biopsy felt, as the needle was inserted, that he had been chosen by God. The moment the delusion occurred can often be described as precisely as this. The delusion cannot be explained, except in terms of a delusional perception, and it is not explained by other members of the subject's cultural and social group. It frequently follows a delusional mood. The experience often results in a delusion of reference or misinterpretation but it may lead to a religious or grandiose or persecutory delusion or to various types of explanatory delusion. The subject must be able to describe this experience precisely and a written account of it must be given. If there is any doubt about the primary nature of the delusion do not rate it here. Always rate the resulting or explanatory delusion as well. Do not include delusions which seem to arise on the basis of a particular mood (e.g. depressive delusions, or grandiose delusions occurring when the patient is elated). Do not, of course, include delusions which are explanations of other phenomena, such as thought insertion, hallucinations, subcultural beliefs, etc. as most are.

It will very rarely be necessary to rate primary delusions as partial since primary delusions enter the mind with full conviction, therefore usually rate (2) if the symptom is present.

83. SUBCULTURALLY INFLUENCED DELUSIONS

Include specific idiosyncratic beliefs held with conviction by small subgroups within the community, e.g. sects, tribes or secret societies, but not by the community at large. If the belief is not elaborated in any way by the subject, and is presented simply as it would be by any other member of the subgroup, rate (1). For example Voodoo, witchcraft or special religious beliefs would come into this category. Do not include widely held religious or superstitious beliefs which are part of the general background of community life and which most people learn in childhood.

If the subculturally derived beliefs mentioned above are held with exceptional fervour and conviction, or are further elaborated by the subject, so that other members of the subgroup might well recognise them as abnormal, rate (2). A subject who elaborated more conventional religious beliefs in an idiosyncratic and delusional way would also be included here. This condition is often the result of excitement, expansiveness, depression, confusion, intellectual retardation, etc., interacting with the subject's beliefs and interests.

If some more recognisable subcultural delusional state is present (Koro, Witigo, etc.), rate (3).

Write down an example to indicate why any positive rating is made.

See note on possession states in definition of symptom 71.

84. MORBID JEALOUSY

The subject, without good reason, thinks that his sexual partner is unfaithful to him. If he is still doubtful about this but cannot help feeling that it might be the case, if he entertains the possibility without actually yielding to conviction, rate (1). If the subject seeks for evidence, interprets innocent patterns of events as proof or makes accusations of unfaithfulness, rate (2).

85. DELUSIONS OF PREGNANCY

The subject thinks she is pregnant although the circumstances make it clear that she cannot possibly be. For example, one subject was a widow, had not had intercourse for several years, was well past the menopause, but was convinced that she had been pregnant for two years. Rate this condition (2) and a partial delusion (1). Always write down an example.

86. SEXUAL DELUSIONS AND HALLUCINATIONS

Any delusion with a sexual content (fantasy lover, sex changing, etc.) other than morbid jealousy (no. 84) or delusion of pregnancy (no. 85) is included here. Rate partial delusions as (1) and full delusional conviction as (2). Write down an example. Include hallucinations.

87. DELUSIONAL MEMORIES, CONFABULATIONS, FANTASTIC DELUSIONS

Delusional memories are experiences of past events which clearly did not occur but which the subject equally clearly remembers, e.g. 'I came down to earth on a silver star in 1964'.

Delusional confabulations are beliefs which the subject can be led on to elaborate during the course of the interview. If the phenomenon is present, however, it usually occurs spontaneously.

Only rate fantastic delusions if the content has not been rated elsewhere (under delusions of paranormal or physical influence, nos. 79 or 80, etc.), e.g. England's coast melting.

Rate partial delusions as (1) and full delusional conviction as (2). Always write down an example.

88. DELUSIONS OF GUILT

This symptom appears to be grounded in a depressed mood. The subject thinks he has brought ruin to his family by being in his present condition or that his symptoms are a punishment for not doing better. He may have a fluctuating awareness that his feelings are an exaggeration of normal guilt. Rate this condition (1). In the more severe form of the symptom, the subject has a delusional conviction that he has sinned greatly, or committed some terrible crime, or brought ruin upon the world; i.e. there may be a grandiose quality to the delusion. He may feel that he deserves punishment, even death or hell-fire, because of it. He may say that his offence and the punishment he has merited are unnameable. Rate this condition (2).

Distinguish from pathological guilt without delusional elaboration, in which the subject is in general aware that the guilt originates within himself and is exaggerated (symptom no. 33).

89. SIMPLE DELUSIONS CONCERNING APPEARANCE

The subject has a strong feeling that something is wrong with his appearance. He looks old or ugly or dead, his skin is cracked, his teeth mishapen, his nose too large or his body crooked. Other people do not notice anything specially wrong but the subject can be reassured only momentarily if at all. There may only be one particular complaint but there is no elaboration of any kind (e.g. if the subject says he has a metal nose, rate symptom 87 not this one). Rate this condition (1).

If the subject has actually acted on the delusion, e.g. has had his teeth out or a plastic operation on his nose, or been to see a surgeon, etc., within past month, rate (2).

Always write down an example.

Exclude selfconsciousness, concern about real skin disease, etc. See symptoms nos. 48 and 90 for differentiation from depersonalisation.

90. DELUSIONS OF DEPERSONALISATION

The subject has a strong feeling as if he had no brain, a hollow within his skull, no thoughts in his head. He can be reassured only temporarily. Rate this condition (1). If the symptom is more intense, the subject has a delusional conviction that he has no head, that he cannot see himself in the mirror, that he has a shadow but no body, that he does not exist at all, rate (2).

Always write down an example.

Exclude delusional elaboration, e.g. that some other force or agency has taken over the subject's mind and body so that he now has another identity and no will of his own (this is symptom no. 71).

91. HYPOCHONDRIACAL DELUSIONS

This symptom is in many ways similar to no. 90, delusions of depersonalisation. The subject feels that his body is unhealthy, rotten or diseased and can only be reassured for a brief while that this is not the case. Rate this condition (1). If the symptom is more intense, so that the subject has a delusional conviction that he has incurable cancer, that his bowels are stopped up or rotting away, rate (2). Always write down an example.

Sometimes it is difficult to decide whether the symptom is 90 or 91, as when the subject says he is hollow and has no inner existence because all his insides have rotted away. In this instance, it is legitimate to rate both symptoms positively. In general, when in doubt rate 91 rather than 90.

92. DELUSIONS OF CATASTROPHE

The subject feels a sense of impending doom, that something awful will happen, but he doesn't know what. He can only be temporarily reassured. The feeling is out of proportion to any possible cause. Rate this condition (1). Affect is usually depressed. If the symptom is more intense, the subject has a delusional conviction that the world is about to end, that some enormous catastrophe has occurred or is going to occur, that the world is decayed, dirty and rotten. Rate this condition (2).

93–6. GENERAL RATINGS OF DELUSIONS AND HALLUCINATIONS

These ratings are self-explanatory.

97. FUGUES, BLACKOUTS, AMNESIAS

The subject complains that there have been periods of at least one hour during the past month (usually longer and possibly lasting days) which he cannot remember at all although he would be expected to remember them in some sort of detail. The subject has no idea where he was nor what he was doing during this time. Do not take possible aetiology into account but simply rate the fact of the amnesia. Rate according to length up to 12 hours (1), 12–24 hours (2), more than 24 hours (3).

98. DRUG ABUSE

Specify any drugs abused during past month other than alcohol. Enter only one category – the highest in the following order: heroin, cocaine (morphine-type); LSD, Amphetamine (amphetamine-hallucinogen type); Amytal (barbiturate-type); cannabis (1).

99. ALCOHOL ABUSE

Specify alcohol abuse during past month according to whether regarded as a problem (1), or whether any item in the check list applies (2).

100. DISSOCIATIVE STATES

A dissociative state is defined as a 'narrowing of consciousness which serves an unconscious purpose and is commonly accompanied or followed by a selective amnesia' (WHO Glossary). Dissociative states associated with alcohol, drugs, epilepsy, etc. are excluded. That is, only include fugues, hypersomnia, trance, etc., if no organic factors are manifest. If present during the past month but not at examination, rate (1). If present at examination, etc. (2). Exclude stupor, which is rated separately as symptom no. 102. See note on possession states in definition of symptom 71.

101. CONVERSION SYMPTOMS

Rate functional symptoms such as paralysis, anaesthesia, blindness, tremor, seizures, etc. Do not include if any clearcut organic cause. If present during the past month but not at examination, rate (1). If present at examination, rate (2).

102. CLOUDING OF CONSCIOUSNESS AND STUPOR

'Clouding of consciousness' is defined as inadequate comprehension of external impressions, with perplexity and impairment of attention and orientation. Rate this condition (1).

'Stupor' is defined as a complete absence, in clear consciousness, of any voluntary movement. Rate this condition (2). Include depressive and 'hysterical' stupor. See note on possession states in definition of symptom 71.

103. ORGANIC IMPAIRMENT OF MEMORY

Three degrees of severity are defined. In the mildest degree, the subject fairly often forgets names or dates or where he put things down or what he intended to do when he initiated a series of actions, and this is uncharacteristic of his past ability to remember. Rate this condition (1). In the second degree of severity, the subject often forgets where he put things, cannot go shopping without a list, sometimes fails to recognise people he knows, will lose his way in an unfamiliar area. Rate this condition (2). In the most severe condition, rate (3), the subject tends to wander if not under supervision because he cannot remember the way, fails to recognise near relatives, does not remember months or seasons.

104. INSIGHT INTO PSYCHOTIC CONDITION

If no psychotic symptoms (from sections 12-15) are present, rate (9). If the subject recognises that the psychotic symptoms are anomalies of his own mental processes, even if he is not very sophisticated about the reasons, rate (0). If he is limited from attaining this degree of understanding only by his level of intelligence or education or social background (which may decree explanations in terms of religion, etc.), rate (1). If he realises that there is something wrong with his mental processes but has a delusional explanation for this (someone is trying to drive him mad, etc.) or if the examiner considers that subject does not accept that his mental processes are affected, in spite of his statements, rate (2). If the subject considers that his mental processes are quite unaffected, whatever other explanation he gives, rate (3).

Always write a note about the degree of insight shown by the patient.

105. INSIGHT INTO NEUROTIC CONDITION

If the subject has psychotic symptoms (sections 12-15), or if he has no neurotic symptoms, rate (9). If he recognises that the neurotic symptoms are anomalies of his own mental processes, even if he is not very sophisticated about the reasons, rate (0). If he is limited from attaining this degree of understanding only by his level of intelligence or education or social background (which may decree explanations of a different kind), rate (1). If he explains neurotic symptoms in physical terms (e.g. palpitations or a backache are regarded as the leading symptoms and thought to be due to heart or vertebral disease), rate (2). If the subject considers that his mental processes are quite unaffected, rate (3).

Always write a note about the degree of insight shown by the subject.

106–7. SOCIAL IMPAIRMENT

These ratings are self-explanatory. They are not symptoms and are used only when no history is available in addition to the PSE.

RATINGS OF BEHAVIOUR

108. SELF-NEGLECT

Consider subject's degree of cleanliness, state of hair, make-up and clothes, whether shaven or not, etc. Only rate self-neglect if there is marked lack of attention to at least one of these aspects of personal appearance: rate this condition (1). If there is marked self-neglect in more than one aspect or if, for example, the subject smells because of self-neglect, rate (2).

Take into account what opportunity the subject has had to take care of his appearance – do not rate self-neglect because the subject is dressed in pyjamas and unshaven, if he has had no chance to look otherwise. Also check whether nursing staff have taken special care to prevent self-neglect from showing (rate 9).

Do not include simple untidiness. Self-neglect must be fairly marked for it to be rated even (1).

109. BIZARRE APPEARANCE

This symptom is only rated on the basis of oddities of appearance which are quite clearly related to the subject's psychotic condition. For example, secret documents or codes, clothes or ornaments with a special significance (one lady wore a specially constructed hat 'to keep the rays off'). Rate (1) or (2) if the whole impression is grossly odd and would be remarked on by a fairly unsophisticated person.

Do not include a mild degree of eccentricity or even a major degree if it is clearly determined by a particular sub-group. The main criterion is whether the odd appearance is determined by the subject's psychotic symptoms.

Do not include mannerisms or posturing which are rated elsewhere (symptom no. 116).

110. SLOWNESS AND UNDERACTIVITY

The subject sits abnormally still or walks abnormally slowly or takes a long time to initiate movement. The symptom has to be fairly marked, and unusual for the subject. Rate (1) if it is not present throughout the interview but there are periods of normal activity or overactivity. Rate (2) if the subject is retarded and underactive throughout the whole interview.

If the retardation or underactivity is thought to be due to medication, rate (9) and specify.

Do not include if retardation is due to organic causes, peripheral or central – rate (9) and specify.

111. AGITATION

This symptom consists of excessive motor movement with a background of marked anxiety. Rate (1) if the subject is markedly fidgety or restless, cannot sit still and is constantly shifting about (a mild degree of this is common and should not be included). Rate (2) if the subject cannot sit in a chair but paces up and down or has to stand up from time to time and possibly break off the interview because of motor restlessness.

Be sure not to include ordinary fidgeting. Agitation is a marked symptom even when rated (1). Distinguish, however, from gross excitement (symptom no. 112) in which the subject runs rather than walks, and is much wilder and perhaps more hostile. Also distinguish from stereotypies (symptom no. 117) in which the subject repeats certain stereotyped movements such as rocking, rubbing, grimacing, etc.

112. GROSS EXCITEMENT AND VIOLENCE

The subject is wildly excited, he runs about the room, jumps, flings his arms about, perhaps shouting or screaming. He may throw things, or be aggressive or destructive. Rate (1) if only one brief episode after which subject calms down and interview can continue. Rate (2) if more than one episode or if more continuous and subject cannot be interviewed because of the symptom.

Distinguish from agitation (symptom no. 111) in which the subject is anxious rather than angry and is not aggressive, destructive or wild.

113. IRREVERENT BEHAVIOUR

The subject sings, makes facetious remarks or silly jokes, is unduly familiar with strangers, does not observe the ordinary social conventions of a medical interview. This behaviour should be marked and unmistakeable, even for a rating of (1). If it is present throughout the interview and affects all situations which arise during it, rate (2). Write down an example.

Distinguish from socially embarrassing behaviour (symptom no. 115).

114. DISTRACTIBILITY

The subject's attention is taken up by trivial events occurring while the interview proceeds which usually would not be noticed, let alone interfere with the interview. The subject may remark on the pattern of the wallpaper instead of replying to a question, or break off to comment on the furniture or the sound of someone walking by. If this is occurring throughout the interview, rate (2). If it occurs quite markedly but not throughout the interview, rate (1). Write down an example.

115. EMBARRASSING BEHAVIOUR

The subject makes sexual suggestions or advances to the interviewer. He does not show social restraint but belches or passes flatus loudly or scratches his genitals or exposes himself, either without shame or without apparent concern for the conventions. If the subject's behaviour is characterised in this way throughout the interview, rate (2). Otherwise rate (1). Write down an example of the subject's behaviour.

Do not include unpolished manners due to lack of social education. Do not include irreverent behaviour (symptom no. 113) but the two symptoms can be present together.

116. MANNERISMS AND POSTURING

Mannerisms are odd, stylised movements or postures, usually specific to the subject often suggestive of special meaning or purpose. The subject may assume or maintain uncomfortable postures for a considerable time. He may salute three times before entering a room or get up and walk round his chair from time to time or make complex gestures with his hands. If the interview is interspersed with mannerisms or postures, rate (2). Otherwise rate (1). Always write down an example.

Do not include stereotypies (symptom no. 117) in which the subject repeats certain stereotyped movements such as rocking, rubbing, nodding or grimacing, but they do not seem to have special significance.

117. STEREOTYPIES AND TICS

The subject performs certain repetitive movements such as rocking to and fro on a chair, rubbing his head round and round with his hand, nodding his head or grimacing. Include tics. These movements do not appear to have any special significance. If they continue more or less throughout the interview, rate (2), otherwise rate (1).

Distinguish from agitation (symptom no. 111) in which the subject is anxious, fidgeting and restless and may pace up and down but does not perform any repetitive movements.

118. BEHAVES AS IF HALLUCINATED BY VOICES

A presumption that the subject is auditorily hallucinated may be made from his behaviour. His lips move soundlessly or he calls out occasionally as though in answer, looking round or up where the voices appear to originate. Be careful with 'giggling to self' which often occurs through embarrassment or shyness and is not necessarily a sign of auditory hallucinations. Distinguish also the champing movements of the mouth which are often present in chronic schizophrenic subjects and those who have been for a long time on phenothiazine drugs.

If the subject appears hallucinated throughout the interview, rate (2), otherwise rate (1).

119. CATATONIC MOVEMENTS

Catatonic movements are nowadays very rare. Do not rate them as present unless there is little doubt about them. *Negativism* occurs when the subject consistently does the opposite of what he is asked, e.g. asked to open his hand he will close it tighter. *Ambitendence* is a fluctuation between two alternatives, e.g. the subject begins to take the hand the examiner proffers him and then withdraws his own hand, and then makes to put it forward again, etc. *Flexibilitas cerea* is a condition in which the muscles of a limb become fairly rigid and the arm, if moved passively, moves without jerking. If an arm is raised into a certain position the patient will hold it for at least fifteen seconds. *Mitgehen* is excessive co-operation in passive movement. The subject can be pushed into uncomfortable postures by finger-tip pressure from the examiner. *Echolalia* is the imitation of words and phrases, using the inflection and tone of voice of the person copied.

If there is suspicion of organic disease, rate (9) and specify.

RATINGS OF AFFECT

120. OBSERVED ANXIETY

The subject has a tense or worried look or posture. He may look and sound fearful or apprehensive. He may have a tremor of voice or hands, a tachycardia, or other evidence of autonomic anxiety. If the subject definitely shows anxiety more or less throughout the interview, rate (2). Otherwise rate (1). Be fairly critical about the threshold of rating. There has to be a fairly marked degree of anxiety present (taking into account that the examination itself may be somewhat anxiety provoking in some subjects) for the symptom to be rated present at all.

121. OBSERVED DEPRESSION

Rate a sad, mournful look with tears in eyes and gloomy monotonous voice, as (1). If subject's voice chokes on distressing topics, he frequently sighs deeply and cries openly, rate (2). Also include 'frozen misery', if examiner is sure that it is present, as (2).

122. HISTRIONIC BEHAVIOUR

The subject's feelings are expressed in an exaggerated, dramatic, histrionic manner. Rate (1) or (2) according to intensity and frequency.

123. HYPOMANIC AFFECT

The subject is moderately elated, unduly smiling and cheerful irrespective of context, but the good humour may readily turn to irritability. Rate this condition (1). If the subject becomes highly elated or exalted rate (2).

124. HOSTILE IRRITABILITY

Rate (1) if the subject is un-cooperative, irritable, prickly, discontented or antagonistic. Rate (2) if he is angry or overtly hostile or if the interview has to be discontinued because of irritability.

Exclude gross excitement (symptom no. 112) – in which the subject becomes wild and may actually attack people or destroy things. The two symptoms can, of course, be present together.

125. SUSPICION

The subject expresses the feeling that everything is not as it should be – this is clear from what he says about his relations with other people and with his environment during the past month. Usually the subject thinks that there may be a deliberate attempt to harm or annoy, beyond what his circumstances would warrant (clearly some people might be suspicious with justification – only pathological suspicion should be rated). If the subject does show suspicion in this sense but is not openly suspicious of the interview procedure, rate (1). If the subject also seems to think that the interviewer, or some part of the interview procedure, is itself part of the process that he suspects is going on, rate (2).

Distinguish from puzzlement, in which the subject does not apparently suspect a particular kind of cause (e.g. a plot or attempt to annoy) but simply does not know how to explain what is going on (symptom no. 126). Remember, however, that some subjects may attempt to conceal the reason for their suspicions.

126. PERPLEXITY

The subject looks puzzled. He cannot make out the explanation for experiences which seem to him unusual. These may be delusions of reference, perceptual changes, intruded thoughts, etc., or the subject may simply be disoriented. Rate (1) or (2) according to the severity and duration of the symptom during the interview.

Perplexity may co-exist with suspicion (symptom no. 125), particularly when the subject does not really know what he is suspicious of, but only that there is something to be suspicious about. The two symptoms are quite separate, however, and should be rated independently.

127. LABILITY OF MOOD

The subject's mood is changeable. At one moment he may be frightened, at another confident. Euphoria may alternate with depression or hostility with friendliness. Include different degrees of manifestation of one mood, e.g. fluctuations between normal cheerfulness and elation. All these variants are included, i.e. consider only the changeability of the mood, not what type of mood is present. Rate (1) or (2) according to the frequency of change and briefness of stable moods.

128. BLUNTED AFFECT

This term includes flatness of affect, emotional indifference and apathy. Essentially, the symptom involves a diminution of emotional response. The subject's face and voice are expressionless, he does not become involved with the interview or respond emotionally to changing topics of conversation, he seems indifferent when apparently distressing matters are discussed (whether or not delusional). There is a very limited range of emotional expression. If severe and fairly uniform throughout the interview, very little rapport, and almost no emotional response, with expressionless face and monotonous voice) - rate (2). If severe but less uniform throughout the interview, or less marked though uniform, rate (1).

Differentiate from incongruity of affect (symptom no. 129), in which affect is expressed but is not in keeping with the affect which would ordinarily be expected.

Make this rating independently of any diagnostic formulation you have in mind (this is true of all ratings in the PSE but particularly of this one). A depressed subject may have a limited range of emotional expression while a schizophrenic subject has a normal range, as well as vice versa.

129. INCONGRUITY OF AFFECT

The range of emotional expression is not necessarily diminished (it may even be increased) but the emotion expressed is not in keeping with that expected. For example, a subject may laugh when discussing a sad event. If this sort of incongruity occurs only a few times during the interview, rate (1). If it occurs more frequently, rate (2).

Do not rate a simple failure to show emotion when expected as incongruity but as blunting (symptom no. 128).

RATINGS OF SPEECH

130. SLOWNESS OF SPEECH

There are long pauses before the subject answers and each word follows very slowly after the one before. Often the subject stops answering altogether and has to be reminded before starting again. The interview may be impossible to complete because the subject is so slow and cannot be hurried. Rate severe slowness, shown throughout the interview, as (2), less marked degrees of the symptom are rated as (1). Always give the subject the benefit of any doubt concerning education, fluency and ability to use language. If in any doubt, rate the symptom as absent.

Differentiate from restricted quantity of speech (symptom no. 134), which is often *not* associated with slowness.

131. PRESSURE OF SPEECH

The subject talks too much, there seems to be undue pressure to get the words out, he speaks too fast, his voice is too loud and unnecessary words are added. If the whole interview is characterised in this way, rate (2). If only parts of the interview are characterised in this way, or if only some of the elements are evident but not others (though the whole impression is definitely abnormal), rate (1).

132. NON-SOCIAL SPEECH

Non-social speech is speech which quite clearly does not fit within the social context of the interview, i.e. which is not addressed to the examiner in answer to questions or as part of the conversation. Irrelevant or incoherent replies to or comments on the examiner's questions are counted as social, not non-social, speech. Include talking, muttering or whispering to self spontaneously or trailing on after a question has been answered, shouting 'to voices', soundless lip-movements, etc. Rate (1) if definitely present but not a marked feature of the interview. Rate (2) if a marked feature of the interview (in which case the interview is likely to be incomplete).

Do not rate non-social speech as present unless it clearly fits the definition. If in doubt, exclude it. Always give the subject the benefit of any doubt concerning education, fluency and ability to use language.

133. MUTENESS

Rate (1) if the subject is almost mute, and says no more than twenty words in answer to questions, including introductory section. (Do not include non-social speech when making a rough assessment of number of words used. A 'mute' subject may talk a lot, outside the context of the interview.)

Rate (2) if the subject utters no more than half a dozen recognisable words in answer to questions throughout the interview.

134. RESTRICTED QUANTITY OF SPEECH

The subject repeatedly fails to answer, questions have to be repeated, answers are restricted to the minimum (often one word, or telegrammatic style). Rate this condition (2). If the subject answers readily enough but only with the minimum necessary number of words, and does not use extra sentences or unprompted additional comments, so that it is extremely difficult to keep a conversation going, rate (1). For example:

Q. 'What work do you do?'

A. 'I'm a machinist. I work at Simpson's.' Pause, then without prompting: 'It's a decent sort of job really.'

'I work at Simpson's' is an extra sentence. 'It's a decent sort of job really' is an unprompted additional comment.

Differentiate from slowness of speech (symptom no. 130) which is usually normal speech slowed down so that the examiner only, in fact, samples rather few words. Restricted quantity does not necessarily imply slowness at all. The two symptoms can, however, appear together.

Always write down an example.

135. NEOLOGISMS AND BIZARRE USE OF WORDS OR PHRASES

Neologisms: words which the subject makes up and which have no generally accepted meaning, e.g. 'Per-God', 'Per-the-Devil', 'tarn-harn'.

Bizarre use of words or phrases: only gross examples, equivalent in their effect to neologisms, should be rated, e.g. 'miracle-willed', 'frequenting of clairvoyance'. Ordinary idiosyncrasies should not be included. Make due allowance for lack of education or intelligence.

Rate (1) if only a few examples. Rate (2) if whole conversation is interlarded with examples.

Always write down the evidence for the rating.

DISORDER OF CONTENT OF SPEECH

Three types of disordered content are specified: incoherence, flight of ideas and poverty. These are overlapping concepts and, in each case, the effect is to make it very difficult to grasp what the subject means. However, the symptoms are defined in terms of specific components so that it should, in most cases, be possible to say whether one, two or all three symptoms are present. If in doubt, rate hierarchically, i.e. rate incoherence in preference to flight of ideas and flight of ideas in preference to poverty of speech.

If the patient does not talk enough to give a rateable sample of speech, rate all three symptoms (9).

136. INCOHERENCE OF SPEECH

The subject's grammar is distorted (e.g. 'They've all been going he she first wife'), or he answers beside the point ('What is the colour of grass?' 'Red'), or he uses grossly pedantic phrases which obscure his meaning, or there are unexplained shifts from topic to topic ('knight's move'), or there is a lack of logical connection between one part of a sentence and another or between one sentence and the next. For example:

We've seen the downfall of the radium crown by the Roman Catholics, whereas when you come to see the drinking side of the business, God saw that Noah, if he lost his reason, he got nobody there to look after them.

I did suggest to you, that intrinsic or congenital sentiment or refinement of disposition would be so miracle-willed through God's 'tarn-harn' as to assume quite the opposite.

I believe we live in a world, in an age, where the elements are a force that elders of professionalism hope, not to conquer, but to control.

If the subject's speech is completely incoherent, as in these three examples, rate (2). A lesser degree of incoherence, so that some of the subject's meaning does get through, is rated (1).

Always make due allowance for poor education, poor intelligence or poor grasp of the language. Always write down an example.

Differentiate from hypomanic content of speech (symptom no. 137) 'flight of ideas' is a movement from one theme to another, which is fairly easy to follow because of clang associations or associations of the white–black–coffin variety. 'Knight's move' is a totally unexpected switch of topic, with no link apparent (or only a sophisticated interpretation can make sense of it). The two symptoms *can* be present together but are very difficult to isolate from each other. It is then best to rate the identifiable component as present and make the other (9).

137. FLIGHT OF IDEAS

Words are associated together inappropriately because of their meaning or rhyme (white–black–coffin, splash–hash–fascist) so that speech loses its aim and the subject wanders far from his original theme. There may also be comments on irrelevant events such as someone sneezing outside the room. There is frequent punning. If the whole conversation is of this kind, so that it is difficult to conduct a useful interview at all, rate (2). If flight of ideas is marked but it is still possible to grasp some of the subject's meaning, rate (1). Always write down a sample of the speech.

Differentiate from 'knight's move' in which it is very difficult to see how the change in topic comes about (symptom no. 136).

138. POVERTY OF CONTENT OF SPEECH

The subject talks fairly freely but so vaguely that no information is given, in spite of the number of words used. This symptom may appear to be readily recognisable in some of one's colleagues, therefore only rate it when it is really pathological. The following example would be rated (2).

Q. 'How do you like it in hospital?'

A. 'Well, er ... not quite the same as, er ... don't know quite how to say it. It isn't the same, being in hospital as, er ... working, er ... the job isn't quite the same, er ... very much the same but, of course, it isn't exactly the same.'

Include also examples of frequent repetitiveness or blocking ('sudden interruption in a line of speech without recognisable reason, so that the subject stops in the middle of a sentence and cannot recapture the theme') or perseveration. These would usually be rated as (1).

Always make due allowance for poor education or intelligence or use of language. Always write down a sample of speech by way of example.

139. MISLEADING ANSWERS

The subject answers at random, or answers 'yes' to all questions, or frequently contradicts himself, or appears to be deliberately misleading. If marked, so that it is difficult to trust any of the ratings made, rate (2). If only some of the replies seem to be misleading, rate (1).

140. ADEQUACY OF INTERVIEW

This has already been rated following the introductory part of the interview. Rerate, taking into account all the subject's replies and the circumstances of the interview.

PRESENT STATE EXAMINATION
(Ninth edition of interview schedule, May 1973)

© Medical Research Council 1974

Project no.

	1	2

Subject no.

	3	4	5

Card no.

	6	7

	8	9	10

Interviewed at:

Interviewed by:

Date and time of interview:

Type of service or setting:

Date of admission, etc.:

Name of agency:

Interview rated by:

Date of rating:

Live _____ V/T _____ A/T _____ Film _____

Episode no.

MRC Social Psychiatry Unit
Institute of Psychiatry
London
SE5 8AF

INSTRUCTIONS

The instruction manual contains a detailed description of the origins, development and underlying principles of the PSE and a glossary of definitions of symptoms. The examiner must be thoroughly familiar with the manual and glossary and should have had some prior training in the use of the PSE.

Four kinds of question are written into the schedule:

(a) Obligatory (starred) questions

These must be asked if the interview is conducted at all. Only 54 questions are involved. Thus subjects with no symptoms, who ask clarifying questions of their own and who answer clearly and decisively, can be screened very quickly indeed. Whenever there is any doubt, however, and certainly whenever a symptom needs clarification, the second kind of question should be asked.

(b) Bracketed questions above cut-off points

These help to define the nature and extent of a symptom and should always be asked if there is any doubt about replies to obligatory questions.

(c) Unbracketed questions below cut-off points

Once the examiner has proceeded below a cut-off point, he must ask *all* the unbracketed questions in that part of the section.

(d) Bracketed questions below cut-off points

These serve the same function as similar questions above cut-off points, i.e. they help to define the nature and extent of a symptom. They are used only if there is some other evidence that the symptom is present.

In addition, the examiner himself will usually wish to ask other questions which are not written into the schedule, either general probes or more specific questions, depending on the nature of the patient's replies.

Each symptom is defined to some extent within the schedule itself but the examiner must be completely familiar with the fuller definitions in the glossary. A full discussion of scoring is also included in the glossary, particularly as to how to differentiate (0) from (1), and (1) from (2).

(0) = Examiner satisfied that symptom not present to clinically significant degree during past month.

(8) = Examiner not sure whether symptom present during past month, even though the appropriate questions have been asked, and answered without incoherence or evasion. The symptom cannot be excluded.

(9) = No rating can be made because question not asked or subject does not answer or answer is incomprehensible.

It should be emphasised that using the PSE schedule will not in itself guarantee useful results. The quality of the output of any system depends on the quality of the input.

1. INTRODUCTION

The interviewer should introduce himself briefly, describe the purpose of the interview and explain about any recording equipment. The purpose of the introductory section is to obtain an overall picture of the symptomatology, in the subject's own words.

** To begin with, I should like to get an idea of the sort of problems that have been troubling you during the past month. What have been the main difficulties?

Record the main symptoms spontaneously mentioned.

Means of exploration, if subject gives inadequate information:

If subject's statement too brief	Can you tell me more about that?
If subject has no more to add	What else has been troubling you?
If statements are difficult to understand	Can you explain what you mean by . . . ?
If subject is vague	Could you give an example of . . . ?
If no other response forthcoming	Why did you come to the (hospital)?

RATE PATIENT'S ACCOUNT OF SYMPTOMS.

0 = Subject responds adequately.

1 = Account somewhat inadequate but interview can proceed.

2 = Account seriously inadequate but interview proceeds in an attempt to rate some subjective responses, as well as behaviour, affect and speech.   _____
                                                                                                    (see 140)

3 = Impossible to continue with interview. Only behaviour, affect and speech sections rated.

REASONS FOR INADEQUACY (TICK AS MANY AS APPROPRIATE).

Denial or guardedness	_____	Inattention	_____
Incoherence	_____	Refusal	_____
Irrelevance	_____	Patient mute, stuporous, etc.	_____
Replies too brief	_____	Other, specify	_____
Poverty of content of speech	_____		

IF (1) OR (2) CARRY ON WITH SECTION 2, UNLESS SUBJECT MENTIONS OR HINTS AT DELUSIONS OR HALLUCINATIONS → SECTION 18.

Cut off

Current treatment, if subject not seen in hospital or clinic
Rate the following if sufficient information has already emerged.
If not, use the suggested question:
May I ask if you are seeing any doctor for your nerves?
Or specify if psychosomatic complaints.

What kind of doctor is he?
Your own GP? A private doctor? Psychiatrist?
   0 = No doctor
   1 = GP
   2 = Private doctor other than GP
   3 = Psychiatrist
   4 = Hospital out-patient (other than psychiatric)
   5 = Other paramedical specialist, or osteopath
   6 = Other specify

Are you attending for treatment any person who is not medically qualified, e.g. lay therapist, herbalist, acupuncture, faith healer, Christian Science, church which forbids medical advice?
What were you complaining of at the time?

Specify type of treatment

Complaint

2. HEALTH, WORRYING, TENSION

** Is your physical health good?
   (Does your body function normally?)

** Do you feel you are physically ill in any way?
   (What is that like? How serious is it?)

RATE SUBJECT'S OWN SUBJECTIVE EVALUATION OF
PRESENT PHYSICAL HEALTH (*irrespective of whether physical
disease is present*).   ☐ (1)
   0 = Feels physically very fit.
   1 = Feels particular physical complaint but does not say positively feels fit.
   2 = Feels unwell but not seriously incapacitated.
   3 = Feels seriously incapacitated by physical illness.

** What does your doctor say is wrong?
(Have you had a physical illness recently; colds, influenza, etc.?)

RATE PRESENCE OF PHYSICAL ILLNESS OR HANDICAP,
taking results of recent investigations and physical state exami-
nations into account. ☐ (2)

    0 = No physical illness or handicap present.
    1 = Mild but significant physical illness or handicap (e.g. influenza or limp).
    2 = More serious physical illness or handicap present but not incapacitating
        or threatening to life (e.g. deafness or duodenal ulcer).
    3 = Physical illness or handicap present which is incapacitating or threatening
        to life (e.g. blindness or carcinoma).

Specify illness, disabilities and duration:

RATE PSYCHOSOMATIC SYMPTOMS.
Special projects only ☐ (3)

** Have you worried a lot during the past month?
(What do you worry about?)
PROBE: (Money, housing, children, health, work, marriage, relatives, friends,
neighbours, other).
(How much do you worry? Are you a worrier?)
If any indication of worry, use further probes:

** What is it like when you worry?
(What sort of state of mind do you get into?)
(Do unpleasant thoughts constantly go round and round in your mind?)
(Can you stop them by turning your attention to something else?)

RATE WORRYING: *A round of painful thought which cannot*
be stopped and is out of proportion to the subject worried about. ☐ (4)

    1 = Symptom definitely present during past month, but of moderate clinical
        intensity or intense less than 50% of the time.
    2 = Symptom clinically intense more than 50% of the month.

** Have you had headaches, or other aches or pains, during the past month?
(What kind?)
RATE ONLY TENSION PAINS, e.g. *'band round head',*
'pressure', 'tightness in scalp', 'ache in back of neck', etc., not
migraine. ☐ (5)

    1 = Symptom definitely present during past month, but of moderate clinical
        intensity, or intense less than 50% of the time.
    2 = Symptom clinically intense more than 50% of past month.

** Have you been getting exhausted and worn out during the day or evening, even
when you haven't been working very hard?
RATE TIREDNESS OR EXHAUSTION: *Do not include*
tiredness due to 'flu, etc. = 9. ☐ (6)

    1 = Only moderate form of symptom (tiredness) present; or intense form
        (exhaustion) less than 50% of the time.
    2 = Intense form of symptom (exhaustion) present more than 50% of the
        past month.

** Have you had difficulty in relaxing during the past month?
(Do your muscles feel tensed up?)

RATE MUSCULAR TENSION: *Do not include a subjective feeling of nervous tension, which is rated later.*

☐ (7)

    1 = Symptom definitely present during past month, but of moderate clinical intensity, or intense less than 50% of the time.

    2 = Symptom clinically intense more than 50% of past month.

** Have you been so fidgety and restless that you couldn't sit still?·
RATE RESTLESSNESS.

☐ (8)

(Do you have to keep pacing up and down?)

    1 = Only moderate form of symptom (fidgety, restless) present; or intense form (pacing, can't sit down) less than 50% of the time.

    2 = Intense form of symptom (pacing, etc.) present more than 50% of past month.

** Do you tend to worry over your physical health?

RATE HYPOCHONDRIASIS: *Overconcern with possibility of death, disease or malfunction. Re-rate at end of interview if subject constantly reverts to hypochondriacal preoccupation. Consider ratings of symptoms (1) and (3).*

☐ (9)

    1 = Symptom present during past month, but not (2).

    2 = Subject constantly reverts to hypochondriacal preoccupations during interview.

** Do you often feel on edge or keyed up or mentally tense or strained?
(Do you generally suffer with your nerves?)
(Do you suffer from nervous exhaustion?)

RATE SUBJECTIVE FEELING OF 'NERVOUS TENSION':
There is no need for autonomic accompaniments for this symptom to be rated present.

☐ (10

    1 = Symptom definitely present during past month, but of moderate intensity, or intense less than 50% of the time.

    2 = Intense form of symptom present more than 50% of the past month.

** Do you find that a lot of noise upsets you?
(Do noises sometimes seem to penetrate, or go through your head?)

RATE HYPERSENSITIVITY TO NOISE.

☐

    1 = Moderate degree during month.

    2 = Severe degree during month.

3. AUTONOMIC ANXIETY

In this section, rate only subjective anxiety with autonomic accompaniments, either free-floating or situational. Do not include worrying or nervous tension. Do not include anxiety due to, e.g., persecutory delusions, except in the special item (no. 13).

(CHECK LIST of autonomic accompaniments:

Blushing	Dry mouth
Butterflies	Giddiness
Choking	Palpitations
Difficulty getting breath	Sweating
Dizziness	Trembling)

** Have there been times lately when you have been very anxious or frightened?
(What was this like?)
(Did your heart beat fast?)   *Ask for other autonomic symptoms.*
(How often in the past month?)
RATE FREE-FLOATING AUTONOMIC ANXIETY: *Exclude if due to delusions. Exclude if purely situational.*   (11)

    1 = Symptom definitely present, with autonomic accompaniment, during past month, but of moderate clinical intensity, or intense less than 50% of the time.
    2 = Symptom clinically intense more than 50% of the time.

** Have you had the feeling that something terrible might happen?
(That some disaster might occur but you are not sure what? Like illness or death or ruination?)
(Have you been anxious about getting up in the morning because you are afraid to face the day?)
(What did it feel like?)
RATE ANXIOUS FOREBODING WITH AUTONOMIC ACCOMPANIMENTS.   (12)

    1 = Symptom definitely present, with autonomic accompaniment, during past month, but of moderate clinical intensity, or intense less than 50% of the time.
    2 = Symptom clinically intense more than 50% of the time.

RATE AUTONOMIC ANXIETY DUE TO DELUSIONS, *etc. and if necessary defer to end of interview.*   (13)

    0 = No anxiety due to delusions or hallucinations.
    1 = Subject complains of anxiety but no evidence of anxiety on examination.
    2 = Clearly anxious or frightened because of delusions or hallucinations.

CUT OFF IF NO EVIDENCE OF ANXIETY OR IF ANXIETY DUE ONLY TO DELUSIONS → SECTION 4.

Cut off

Have you had times when you felt shaky, or your heart pounded, or you felt sweaty, and you simply had to do something about it?
(What was it like?)
(What was happening at the time?)
(How often during the past month?)

RATE PANIC ATTACKS WITH AUTONOMIC SYMPTOMS:
A panic attack is intolerable anxiety leading to some action to end it, e.g. leaving a bus, phoning husband at work, going in to see a neighbour, etc.

1 = One to four panic attacks during month
2 = Panic attacks five times or more.

(14)

Do you tend to get anxious in certain situations, such as travelling, or being alone, or being in a lift or tube train?
(What situations? How often during the past month?)
(CHECK LIST: *Can be presented on separate card and each item rated separately, if needed.*
Crowds (shop, street, theatre, cinema, church).
Going out alone; being at home alone.
Enclosed spaces (hairdresser, phone booth, tunnel).
Open spaces, bridges.
Travelling (buses, cars, trains).)

RATE SITUATIONAL AUTONOMIC ANXIETY.

(15)

1 = Has not been in such situations during the past month but aware that anxiety would have been present if the situation had occurred.
2 = Situation has occurred during the past month and patient did feel anxious because of it.

What about meeting people, e.g. going into a crowded room, making conversation?
(CHECK LIST: *Present card if necessary:*
Speaking to an audience.
Eating, drinking or writing in front of other people.
Parties.)

RATE AUTONOMIC ANXIETY ON MEETING PEOPLE.

(16)

1 = Has not been in such situations during the past month but aware that anxiety would have been present if the situation had occurred.
2 = Situation has occurred during the past month and patient did feel anxious because of it.

Do you have any special fears, like some people are scared of feathers or cats or spiders or birds?
(CHECK LIST: *Present card if necessary:*
Heights, thunderstorms, darkness.
Animals or insects of any kind.
Dentists, injections, blood, injury.)

RATE ONLY SPECIFIC PHOBIAS, NOT GENERAL
SITUATIONAL ANXIETY.   (17)

   1 = Has not been in such situations during the past month but aware that anxiety
      would have been present if the situation had occurred.
   2 = Situation has occurred during the past month and patient did feel anxious
      because of it.

Do you avoid any of these situations (specify as appropriate) because you know you
will get anxious?
(How much does it affect your life?)
RATE AVOIDANCE OF ANXIETY-PROVOKING SITUATIONS.   (18)

   1 = Subject tends to avoid such situations whenever possible.
   2 = Marked generalisation of avoidance has occurred during past month, e.g.
      subject has not dared to leave the house or has gone out only if accompanied.

Describe anxiety symptoms and list phobias.

4. THINKING, CONCENTRATION, ETC.

** Can you think clearly or is there any interference with your thoughts?

** Do your thoughts tend to be muddled or slow?
   (Can you make up your mind about simple things quite easily?) (Make decisions
   about everyday matters?)
   RATE SUBJECTIVELY INEFFICIENT THINKING *(if due to
   intrusion of alien thoughts, rate 9).*   (19)

     1 = Symptom definitely present during the past month, but of moderate
       clinical intensity, or intense less than 50% of the time.
     2 = Symptom clinically intense more than 50% of the past month.

** What has your concentration been like recently?
   (Can you read an article in the paper or watch a TV programme right through?)
   (Do your thoughts drift off so that you don't take things in?)

   RATE POOR CONCENTRATION.   (20)

     1 = Only moderate form of symptom present during the past month (e.g. can
       read a short article, can concentrate if tries hard); or intense less than
       50% of the time.
     2 = Symptom clinically intense (cannot attempt to read or concentrate)
       more than 50% of the past month.

** Do you tend to brood on things?
   (So much that you even neglect your work?)
   RATE NEGLECT DUE TO BROODING.   (21)

     1 = Symptom has caused moderate impairment to work or social
       relationships.
     2 = Marked impairment.

** What about your interests, have they changed at all?
(Have you lost interest in work, or hobbies, or recreations?)
(Have you let your appearance go?)

RATE LOSS OF INTEREST *continuing during the past month.* ▢ (22)

    1 = Symptom definitely present during the past month, but of moderate
        clinical severity or severe loss less than 50% of the time.
    2 = Symptom clinically severe more than 50% of the past month.

** Have you become interested in new things at all?

IF EVIDENCE OF EXPANSIVE MOOD OR IDEAS → SECTION 9.

IF ODD IDEAS, EXPLORE FURTHER. PROCEED TO SECTION 15
IF APPROPRIATE.

** Have you suffered any lapses of memory recently? (PROBE ONLY)

IF EVIDENCE OF DISSOCIATION OR ORGANIC MEMORY LOSS →
SECTION 16.

ANSWERS TO THESE QUESTIONS MAY SUGGEST THAT OTHER TYPES
OF THOUGHT DISORDER ARE PRESENT, IF NOT, CUT OFF →
SECTION 5.

—————————————————————————| Cut off |▢|—————

IF ANY EVIDENCE OF THOUGHT DISORDER:

Are you in full control of your thoughts?
Can people read your mind?
Is anything like hypnotism or telepathy going on?

IF NECESSARY, PROCEED TO SECTION 13.

5. DEPRESSED MOOD

** Do you keep reasonably cheerful or have you been very depressed or low-
spirited recently?
Have you cried at all?
(When did you last really enjoy doing anything?)

RATE DEPRESSED MOOD. N.B. *When rating clinical severity
of depression remember that deeply depressed people may not* ▢ (23)
necessarily cry. See definition in glossary.

    1 = Only moderately depressed during past month, or deep depression for
        less than 50% of the time and tending to vary in intensity.
    2 = Deeply depressed for more than 50% of the past month, and tending to
        be unvarying in intensity.

** How do you see the future?
(Has life seemed quite hopeless?)
(Can you see any future?)
(Have you given up or does there still seem some reason for
trying?)
RATE HOPELESSNESS *on subject's own view at present.*

□ (24)

1 = Hopelessness of moderate intensity but still has some degree of hope for
the future (irrespective of time during month).
2 = Intense form of symptom (patient has given up hope altogether).

USE JUDGEMENT ABOUT WORDING.

** Have you felt that life wasn't worth living?
(Did you ever feel like ending it all?)
(What did you think you might do?)
(Did you actually try?)
RATE SUICIDAL PLANS OR ACTS.

□ (25)

1 = Deliberately considered suicide (not just a fleeting thought) but made no
attempt.
2 = Suicidal attempt but subject's life never likely to be in serious danger,
except unintentionally.
3 = Suicidal attempt apparently designed to end in death (i.e. accidental
discovery or inefficient means).

N.B. *Examiner should judge clinically whether there was intent to end life or
not. If in doubt, assume not.*

―――――――――――――――――――――――――| Cut off |――――――

IF EVIDENCE OF BOTH DEPRESSION AND ANXIETY RATE
ANXIETY OR DEPRESSION PRIMARY.

*If subject suffers from both anxiety and depression, and both have been rated as
present, try to decide which is primary.*
Which seems worse, the depression or the anxiety? (Use patient's own terms).

0. Anxiety is primary. Depression appears to be entirely explicable
in terms of the limitations placed on the subject by the symptoms of anxiety, e.g. being unable to leave the house, travel,
meet people, etc., or being afraid of heart disease because of
palpitations.

□ (26)

1. Anxiety and depression both present but seem independent of each other or
it is not possible to decide whether one of them is primary.
2. Depression is primary. Anxiety is either a result of the depression (e.g. subject
is frightened because of morbid or suicidal ideas) or it takes the form of fears
of catastrophe, forebodings about illness or death, dread of having to face the
day when first waking in the morning, preoccupation that something awful is
going to happen. Panic attacks and situational anxiety, if present, are
secondary to depression

Is the depression worse at any particular time of day?
RATE MORNING DEPRESSION *(particularly on waking)*   (27)

  0 = No depression.
  1 = Not specially marked in mornings.
  2 = Specially marked in mornings.

6. SELF AND OTHERS

** Have you wanted to stay away from other people?
   (Why?)
   (Have you been suspicious of their intentions? Of actual harm?)
   RATE SOCIAL WITHDRAWAL.   (28)

   1 = Only passive form of symptom, i.e. subject does not seek company but
       does not refuse it if offered; or, if active withdrawal, less than 50% of
       the month.
   2 = Actively avoids company (refuses it if offered). Actively withdraws in
       this way for more than 50% of the month.

** What is your opinion of yourself compared to other people?
   (Do you feel better, or not as good, or about the same as most?)
   (Do you feel inferior or even worthless?)
   RATE SELF-DEPRECIATION.   (29)

   1 = Some inferiority, not amounting to feeling of worthlessness. If subject
       considers self to be worthless, this intense form of the symptom is
       present less than 50% of the time.
   2 = Subject considers self to be completely worthless. Symptom present
       more than 50% of the month.

** How confident do you feel in yourself:
   (For example, in talking to others, or in managing your relations with other
   people?)
   RATE LACK OF SELF-CONFIDENCE WITH OTHER
   PEOPLE. *Consider only competence in social relationships, not
   competence at mechanical work, etc.*   (30)

   1 = Moderate lack of self-confidence, or intense lack less than 50% of the
       month.
   2 = Intense lack of self-confidence more than 50% of the month.

** Are you self-conscious in public?
   (Do you get the feeling that other people are taking notice of you in the street
   or a bus or a restaurant?)
   (Do they ever seem to laugh at you or talk about you critically?)
   (Do you consider people really are looking at you, or is it
   perhaps the way you feel about it?)
   RATE SIMPLE IDEAS OF REFERENCE (NOT DELUSIONS).   (31)

   1 = Marked self-consciousness only (irrespective of time during month).
   2 = Feels that people are criticising or laughing at self but can be reassured.

IF NO EVIDENCE OF GUILT, CUT OFF → SECTION 7.

(IF EVIDENCE OF MISINTERPRETATIONS, DELUSIONS OF REFERENCE OR PERSECUTION → SECTIONS 15 B, 15 C.)

———————————————————————| Cut off | |——————

IF EVIDENCE OF GUILT:

Do you have the feeling that you are being blamed for something, or even accused? What about?
RATE GUILTY IDEAS OF REFERENCE. *Do not include justifiable*   ☐ (32)
blame or accusation. Exclude delusions of guilt.

    1 = Subject feels blamed but not accused (irrespective of time during month).
    2 = Subject feels accused of some sin or misdemeanour. Not delusional

IF DELUSIONS OF REFERENCE MAY BE PRESENT → SECTION 15 B.

Do you tend to blame yourself at all?
(If people are critical, do you think you deserve it?)   ☐ (33)
RATE PATHOLOGICAL GUILT ONLY.

    1 = Subject feels over-guilty about some peccadillo (irrespective of time during month).
    2 = Subject feels to blame for everything that has gone wrong even when not his fault, but not delusional.

IF DELUSIONS OF GUILT MAY BE PRESENT → SECTION 15 G.

Do you blame anyone else for your troubles?

IF DELUSIONS OF PERSECUTION → SECTION 15 C.

7. APPETITE, SLEEP, RETARDATION, LIBIDO

** What has your appetite been like recently?
    (Have you lost any weight during the past three months?)
    RATE LOSS OF WEIGHT DUE TO POOR APPETITE.   ☐ (34)
    Do not include changes due to physical illness.

    1 = Less than 7 lb (15 kg).
    2 = 7 lb (15 kg) or more.

** Have you had any trouble getting off to sleep during the past month?
    (How long do you lie awake?)
    (What happens if you take sleeping tablets?)
    (How often does it happen?)

RATE DELAYED SLEEP.   □ (35)
   1 = One hour or more delay (irrespective of sleeping tablets).
   2 = Two hours or more delay (irrespective of sleeping tablets).
      (In either case, ten or more nights during month.)

** Do you seem to be slowed down in your movements, or to have too little
   energy recently? How much has it affected you?
   (Do things seem to be moving too fast for you?)
   RATE SUBJECTIVE ANERGIA AND RETARDATION.   □ (36)
   1 = Marked subjective listlessness and lack of energy.
   2 = Marked retardation and underactivity (Irrespective of time during month).

   IF NO APPETITE OR SLEEP DISTURBANCE, AND NO DEPRESSION,
   CUT OFF → SECTION 8.

   ──────────────────────────────────── Cut off │   │ ──

IF SLEEP DISTURBANCE OR DEPRESSION:

Do you wake early in the morning?
RATE EARLY WAKING *(one hour before usual)*.   □ (37)
   1 = One hour or more before ordinary time.
   2 = Two hours or more before ordinary time.
      (In either case, ten or more nights during month.)

Has there been any change in your interest in sex?
RATE LOSS OF LIBIDO WITHIN PRESENT EPISODE OF
ILLNESS AND PERSISTING DURING PAST MONTH.   □ (38)
   1 = Marked loss of interest and performance.
   2 = Almost total loss of libido.

Does the depression or tension get worst just before the start of the monthly
period?

RATE PREMENSTRUAL EXACERBATION   □ (39)
   0 = No definite exacerbation.
   1 = Marked exacerbation.

8. IRRITABILITY

** Have you been very much more irritable than usual recently?
   (How do you show it?)
   (Do you keep it to yourself, or shout, or even hit people?)
   RATE IRRITABILITY.   □ (40)
   1 = Keeps irritation to himself.
   2 = Shows anger by shouting or quarrelling.
   3 = Shows anger by hitting people, throwing or breaking things.

9. EXPANSIVE MOOD AND IDEATION

** Have you sometimes felt particularly cheerful and on top of the world, without any reason?
(Too cheerful to be healthy?)
(How long does it last?)
RATE EXPANSIVE MOOD: *not ordinary high spirits.*

☐ (41)

> 1 = Moderately expansive mood (euphoria with marked element of inappropriateness or excitement, whether recognised by subject or not), present during past month, and persistent for hours at a time.* *Do not include transient high spirits.* Not necessarily described by subject.
>
> 2 = Intense form of symptom (elation or exaltation) definitely present during past month and persistent for hours at a time. Described by subject.

** Have you felt particularly full of energy lately, or full of exciting ideas?
(Do things seem to go too slowly for you?)
(Do you need less sleep than usual?)
(Do you find yourself extremely active but not getting tired?)
(Have you developed new interests recently?)
RATE SUBJECTIVE IDEOMOTOR PRESSURE.

☐ (42)

> 1 = Subjective equivalent of flight of ideas. Images and ideas flash through the mind, each suggesting others, at a faster rate than usual. State persists for hours at a time.* Definitely occurred during past month.
>
> 2 = As (1) but accompanied by very high energy output and activity which does not seem to make subject tired at the time. Definitely occurred during past month and persisted for hours at a time.*

IF NO EVIDENCE OF EXPANSIVE MOOD AND IDEATION, CUT OFF →
SECTION 10.

—————————————————————————————| Cut off | |——————

IF EVIDENCE OF EXPANSIVE MOOD AND IDEATION:

Have you seemed super-efficient at work, or as though you had special powers or talents quite out of the ordinary?
Have you felt specially healthy?
Have you been buying any interesting things recently?
RATE GRANDIOSE IDEAS AND ACTIONS.

☐ (43)

> 1 = Subjective feeling of superb health, exceptionally high intelligence, extraordinary abilities, etc. Persistent for hours at a time.* Symptom occurred at some time during the month.
>
> 2 = Grandiose ideas have been translated into action during the month, e.g. overspending, gambling, etc., under the influence of grandiose ideas and expansive affect. *Do not include compulsive gambling unless clearly of this type.*

(→ GRANDIOSE DELUSIONS, SECTION 15 D IF NECESSARY.)

* *If symptom was more transient but very intense or frequently repeated, it may still be included.*

10. OBSESSIONS

These symptoms are usually experienced as occurring against conscious resistance (see definition in glossary).

** Do you find that you have to keep on checking things that you know you have already done?
(Like gas taps, doors, switches, etc.)
(Do you have to touch or count things many times or repeat the same action over and over again?)
(What happens when you try to stop?)
RATE OBSESSIONAL CHECKING AND REPEATING.   □ (44

  1 = Symptom of moderate intensity or, if severe, present less than 50% of the time.
  2 = Symptom present in severe degree, more than 50% of the past month.

** Do you spend a lot of time on personal cleanliness, like washing over and over even though you know you are clean? What about tidiness?
(Do you get worried by contamination with germs?)
(Do you have other rituals?)
(What happens when you try to stop?)
RATE OBSESSIONAL CLEANLINESS AND SIMILAR RITUALS.   □ (45

  1 = Symptom of moderate intensity or, if severe, present less than 50% of the time.
  2 = Symptom present in severe degree, more than 50% of the past month.

** Do you find it difficult to make decisions even about trivial things?
(Do you constantly have to question the meaning of the universe?)
(Do you get awful thoughts coming into your mind even when you try to keep them out?)
(What happens when you try to stop?)
RATE OBSESSIONAL IDEAS AND RUMINATION.   □ (46

  1 = Symptom of moderate intensity or, if severe, present less than 50% of the time.
  2 = Symptom present in severe degree, more than 50% of the past month.

11. DEREALISATION AND DEPERSONALISATION

** Have you had the feeling recently that things around you were unreal?
(As though everything was an imitation of reality, like a stage set, with people acting instead of being themselves?)
(What is it like? How do you explain it?)
RATE DEREALISATION.   □ (47

  1 = Moderately intense form of symptom definitely occurred during the past month, and persisted for hours at a time. Things appear colourless and artificial, people appear lifeless and seem to act rather than being themselves.

2 = Intense form of symptom occurred during the past month and persisted for hours at a time, e.g. whole world appears like a gigantic stage set, with imitation instead of real objects and puppets instead of people. (If delusional, do not rate here but symptom 90.)

** Have you yourself felt unreal, that you were not a person, not in the living world?
(Or that you were outside yourself, looking at yourself from outside?)
(Or that you look unreal in the mirror?)
(Or that some part of your body did not belong to you?)
(How do you explain it?)
RATE DEPERSONALISATION

(48)

1 = Moderately intense form of the symptom definitely occurred during the past month and persisted for hours at a time. Subject feels himself unreal, a sham, a shadow.
2 = Intense form of symptom definitely occurred during the past month and persisted for hours at a time. Subject feels he is dead, not a person, living in a parallel existence, a hollow shell, even that he does not exist. (If delusional, do not rate here but symptom 90.)

12. OTHER PERCEPTUAL DISORDERS (NOT HALLUCINATIONS)

** Do you ever get the feeling that something odd is going on which you can't explain?
(Or that familiar surroundings seem strange? How do you explain it?)
RATE DELUSIONAL MOOD: *The subject feels that his familiar environment has changed in a way which puzzles him and which he may not be able to describe clearly. The feeling often accompanies delusion formation.*

(49)

1 = Symptom definitely present. No delusions have actually been formulated, though patient may feel that various delusional explanations are possible.
2 = Full delusional elaboration has occurred.

** Does your imagination sometimes play tricks on you?

** Is there anything unusual about the way things look or sound, or smell, or taste?
(Does your body function normally?)
(Is your own appearance normal?)

CONTINUE BELOW CUT-OFF IF NECESSARY, EVEN IF (49) NOT PRESENT.

IF NO PERCEPTUAL ABNORMALITY → SYMPTOM 54.

—————————————————————————————| Cut off | |—————

IF THERE IS ANY HINT OF PERCEPTUAL ABNORMALITY, CONTINUE
BEYOND CUT-OFF POINT AND ALSO CONSIDER LATER SECTIONS.
RATE ONLY BASIC EXPERIENCE, NOT DELUSIONAL ELABORATION.

In what way? Do sounds seem unnaturally clear or loud, or things look vividly
coloured or detailed?
(How do you explain this?)
RATE HEIGHTENED PERCEPTION: *e.g. subject intensely aware
of cracks in a wall, details of a wallpaper pattern, colours in a picture.
Sounds heard with exceptional clarity, music appears particularly
beautiful.*   (50)

> 1 = Subject unable to describe the symptom precisely, but examiner thinks it is
>   likely to have been present at some time during the past month.
> 2 = Subject describes symptom. Definitely present at some time (even if only
>   briefly) during the past month.

Do things seem dark or grey or colourless?
(How do you explain it?)
RATE DULLED PERCEPTION: *The reverse of symptom (50).
Things look, sound and taste dull, flat, colourless and uninteresting.*   (51)

> 1 = Subject unable to describe the symptom precisely, but examiner thinks it is
>   likely to have been present at some time during the past month.
> 2 = Subject describes symptom. Definitely present at some time (even if only
>   briefly) during the past month.

Does the appearance of things or people change in a puzzling way: e.g. distorted
shapes or size or colour?
(How do you explain it?)
RATE CHANGED PERCEPTION.   (52)

> 1 = Subject unable to describe the symptom precisely, but examiner thinks it is
>   likely to have been present at some time during the past month.
> 2 = Subject describes symptom. Definitely present at some time (even if only
>   briefly) during the past month.

Do you think your own appearance is normal?
(Conviction that nose is too large, teeth misshapen, body crooked, etc. Ask
questions here if convenient but rate symptom (89).)

Does your experience of time seem to have changed?
(Does it go too fast or too slowly, or do you seem to live through experiences
exactly as you have had them before?)
RATE CHANGED PERCEPTION OF TIME, INCLUDING
DEJA VU.   (53)

> 1 = Subject unable to describe the symptom precisely, but examiner thinks it is
>   likely to have been present at some time during the past month.
> 2 = Subject describes symptom. Definitely present at some time (even if only
>   briefly) during the past month.

Do you feel you have lost your emotions in some way?
(That you are empty of all feeling, incapable of reacting emotionally?)
(Is this a definite change, or have you always been like that?)
(How do you explain it?)

RATE LOST EMOTIONS: *Rate only subjective loss of affect,
i.e. subject can remember being able to react emotionally, though
this might have been months or even years ago.*   (54)

> 1 = Symptom definitely present during the past month but less than 50% of
> the time.
> 2 = Symptom present more than 50% during the past month.

13. THOUGHT READING, INSERTION, ECHO, BROADCAST

IF QUESTION HAS NOT BEEN COVERED IN SECTION 4 ASK:

** Can you think quite clearly or is there any interference with your thoughts?
(Are you in full control of your thoughts?)
(Can people read your mind?)
(Is anything like hypnotism or telepathy going on?)

IF NO EVIDENCE OF THOUGHT READING, etc., CUT OFF →
SECTION 14.

Cut off

IF ANY EVIDENCE, ASK QUESTIONS BELOW:

*(These symptoms are often recorded as false positives. The examiner must be satis-
fied that the subject is not simply assenting to a question he does not understand,
but genuinely recognises the experience and can describe it so that the examiner
recognises it.) It is particularly important to know the relevant sections of the
Instruction Manual well before rating these symptoms.*

Are thoughts put into your head which you know are not your own?
(How do you know they are not your own?)
(Where do they come from?)

RATE THOUGHT INSERTION: *Include only thoughts recognised
as alien. Do not include delusional elaboration, only basic experience.
(Exclude hallucinations.)*   (55)

> 1 = Symptom described clearly, but subject thinks it may be due to 'own
> unconscious thoughts' etc., i.e. not certainly alien.
> 2 = Symptom described clearly and thoughts described as alien, i.e. inserted into
> mind from elsewhere (even if subject does not know from where). Not
> hallucinations.

Do you ever seem to hear your own thoughts spoken aloud in your head, so that
someone standing near might be able to hear them?
(Are your thoughts broadcast, so that other people know what you are thinking?)
(How do you explain it?)

RATE THOUGHT BROADCAST.   [ ] (56)

    1 = Hears own thoughts 'spoken' aloud but not broadcast. Subject must really hear them aloud in his head. If in doubt rate (8) or (0).

    2 = Thoughts transferred or broadcast so that others can share subject's thoughts even when they are not in the same room. (Do not include 'thoughts being read' unless this is an explanation of thought broadcast. The subject must actually experience his thoughts being available to others.)

Do you ever seem to hear your own thoughts repeated or echoed?
(What is that like? How do you explain it?)
(Where does it come from?)
RATE THOUGHT ECHO OR COMMENTARY.   [ ] (57)

    1 = Thought echo. If any doubt, rate (8) or (0).·

    2 = Subject experiences alien thoughts related to his own thoughts, i.e. associations or comments on his own thoughts. Not hallucinations.

Do you ever experience your thoughts stopping quite unexpectedly so that there are none left in your mind, even when your thoughts were flowing freely before?
(What is that like?)
(How often does it occur? What is it due to?)

Do your thoughts ever seem to be taken out of your head, as though some external person or force were removing them?
(Can you give an example?)
(How do you explain it?)
RATE THOUGHT BLOCK OR WITHDRAWAL.   [ ] (58)

    1 = Thought block. Do not include if due to anxiety or lack of concentration; only if it occurs totally unexpectedly when thoughts are flowing freely. One single occasion is not sufficient for rating. *Be very critical in rating this symptom.*

    2 = Delusional explanation that thoughts are withdrawn.

Can anyone read your thoughts?
(How do you know? How do you explain it?)
RATE DELUSION OF THOUGHTS BEING READ: *Only if subject does not mean that people can infer his thoughts from his actions. (Do not include subject reading thoughts of other people → 76.)*   [ ] (59)

    1 = 'Partial' delusion. Subject entertains the possibility that thoughts might be read but is not certain about it. Exclude if subcultural explanation.

    2 = Full delusion. Exclude if subcultural explanation. The term 'thought reading' is commonly used to mean the ability to tell what someone is thinking from the way they behave – this use should be excluded.

14. HALLUCINATIONS

USE JUDGEMENT ABOUT WORDING.

** I should like to ask you a routine question which we ask of everybody. Do you ever seem to hear noises or voices when there is no one about, and nothing else to explain it?
(Do you ever seem to hear your name being called?)

** Is that true of visions or other unusual experiences, which some people have? (Touch, taste, smell, temperature, pain, etc.)

IF NO EVIDENCE FOR HALLUCINATIONS OF ANY SENSE, CUT OFF →
SECTION 15.

| Cut off |

IF EVIDENCE FOR NON-AUDITORY HALLUCINATIONS ONLY →
SUBSECTIONS 14B and 14C

14A. AUDITORY HALLUCINATIONS

IF ANY EVIDENCE THAT AUDITORY HALLUCINATIONS MIGHT BE PRESENT:

Do you hear noises like tapping, or music? (What is it like?)
Does it sound like muttering or whispering?
Can you make out the words?
RATE NON-VERBAL AUDITORY HALLUCINATIONS.   (60)

   1 = Music, tapping, car engines, etc. Do not include tinnitus.
   2 = Muttering, whispering but subject cannot make out any words at all.

What does the voice say?
(Write down examples of typical verbal hallucinations.)
(If accusatory: Do you think that it is justified? Do you deserve it?)
Do you hear your name being called?
RATE VERBAL HALLUCINATIONS BASED ON DEPRESSION   (61)
OR ELATION OR VOICE CALLING SUBJECT.
*Content is congruent with mood; e.g. 'He's dirty', in context of depression, or
'Go to Westminster', in elated subject who thinks he is Prime Minister. Include
voice calling subject (e.g. calling name) or saying single words only. Be careful to
distinguish from delusions of reference in which people whom the subject can see
are thought to be talking about him.*
RECORD EXAMPLES.

   1 = Voice calling name, or single words only.
   2 = Other verbal hallucinations; congruent with depressed mood.
   3 = Other verbal hallucinations; congruent with elated mood.

Do you hear several voices talking about you?
Do they refer to you as 'he' (she)?
(What do they say?)
(Do they seem to comment on what you are thinking, or reading, or doing?)

RATE VOICE(S) DISCUSSING SUBJECT IN THIRD PERSON
OR COMMENTING ON THOUGHTS OR ACTIONS (NOT
BASED ON DEPRESSION OR ELATION).   ☐ (62)

*Do not include muttering or whispering if subject cannot make out words. Exclude
'dissociative' hallucinations (symptom 64). Do not include voice calling name or
affectively based verbal hallucinations (symptom 61). There may be one voice
commenting on subject's thoughts or actions, or several voices discussing the subject in the third person.*

RECORD EXAMPLES.

 1 = Hears a voice or voices commenting on thoughts or actions in third person
    (e.g. 'Now he's going to go to bed' or 'Why would he think a thing like
    that?'). (2) not present.
 2 = Hears voices talking about him/her in third person (e.g. 'I think he's a homo-
    sexual, don't you?' 'Yes, he wears a pink pullover, that's a sign of it.').
    (1) may also be present.

Do they speak directly to you?
(Are they threatening or unpleasant?)
(Do they call you names?)
Do they give orders? (Do you obey?)

RATE VOICE(S) SPEAKING TO SUBJECT (NOT BASED ON   ☐ (63)
DEPRESSION OR ELATION).

*Include voice(s) speaking directly to subject, whether accusing, threatening, giving
orders or giving information. Exclude voice(s) calling name or based on depression
or elation (symptom 61), or commenting on subject's thoughts or actions
(symptom 62). Exclude 'dissociative' hallucinations (symptom 63).*

RECORD EXAMPLES.

 1 = Pleasant, supportive or neutral voice(s), not based on affect. No hostile
    voices.
 2 = Hostile, threatening or accusing voice(s), thought to be undeserved and not
    based on affect.

N.B. If single isolated words, even with neutral affect, include under 61 (1).

Can you carry on a two-way conversation with —?
(You can reply, and then — replies to you, and you reply again, just as in an
ordinary conversation?)
(Do you see anything, or smell anything at the same time as you hear the voice?)
(Who is it you are talking to?)
(What is the explanation?)
(Do you know anyone else who has this kind of experience?)

RATE 'DISSOCIATIVE' HALLUCINATIONS (VERBAL   ☐ (64)
AND/OR OTHER)

*The subject can hold a two-way conversation with a presence (variously described
as a person, ghost, spirit, god, etc.) which may also be sensed in other ways, e.g.
visually or by touch or smell. Often connected with people with whom the subject
has had strong affective ties. Visual hallucinations can occur alone. There is usually
a strong subcultural colouring, e.g. the subject belongs to a religious sect or to a
subcultural group which sanctions hallucinatory experiences, or the subject has been
under the influence of someone who is involved with such practices. Exclude
hypnogogic hallucinations.*

RECORD EXAMPLES.

    1 = 'Dissociative' hallucinations present. Subject belongs to subcultural group
      or sect in which such experiences are sanctioned.

    2 = 'Dissociative' hallucinations present. Subject does not belong to subcultural
      group as in (1). If not known, rate (1).

Are these voices in your mind or can you hear them through your
ears?
Scoring: (65)

    1 = Subject hears both pseudo-hallucinations (within mind) and true hallucina-
      tions (through ears).

    2 = Subject hears pseudo-hallucinations only.

    3 = Subject hears true hallucinations only.

How do you explain the voice?
RECORD EXPLANATION.

14B. VISUAL HALLUCINATIONS

IF QUESTION HAS NOT BEEN COVERED IN SECTION 12 OR 14A, ASK:

** Have you had visions, or seen things other people couldn't see?

    IF NO EVIDENCE, HERE OR ELSEWHERE, FOR VISUAL
    HALLUCINATIONS CUT OFF → SECTION 15.

——————————————————————————| Cut off |——————

IF ANY EVIDENCE OF VISUAL HALLUCINATIONS:

With your eyes or in your mind?
What did you see?
Were you half asleep at the time?
Has it occurred when you were fully awake?
Did you realise you were 'seeing things'?
Did the vision seem to arise out of a pattern on the wallpaper or a shadow?
How do you explain it?

RATE VISUAL HALLUCINATIONS: *in clear consciousness including pseudo-hallucinations. Exclude 'dissociative' visual hallucinations (symptom 64).*   (66)

   1 = Formless visual hallucinations – flashes of light, shadows, etc.

   2 = Formed visual hallucinations – people, objects like a 'fiery cross', faces, etc.

RATE DELIRIOUS VISUAL HALLUCINATIONS.   (67)

14C. OTHER HALLUCINATIONS

IF QUESTIONS HAVE NOT BEEN COVERED IN PREVIOUS SECTIONS:

** Is there anything unusual about the way things feel, or taste, or smell?

** Does your body function normally?

   IF NO EVIDENCE FOR OTHER HALLUCINATIONS CUT OFF →
   SECTION 15 A.

Cut off

IF ANY EVIDENCE FOR OTHER HALLUCINATIONS:

Do you sometimes notice strange smells that other people don't notice?
(What sort of thing?)
(How do you explain it?)

RATE OLFACTORY HALLUCINATIONS: *Exclude delusion that patient himself smells.*   (68)

   1 = Simple olfactory hallucination. Not delusionally elaborated. Subject smells oranges, death, a burnt smell, scent, etc., which other people cannot smell. Can offer no explanation.

   2 = Delusional elaboration in addition, e.g. gas being put into room.

Do you seem to think that you yourself give off a smell which is noticed?
(What is the explanation?)

RATE DELUSION THAT SUBJECT SMELLS: *Do not include simple preoccupation with body odour, e.g. in anxious subject who sweats a lot.*   (69)

   1 = Subject irrationally thinks he gives off a smell but is not certain. Not sure that others have noticed it but thinks it possible.

   2 = Subject sure that he gives off a smell and that others have noticed it and react accordingly.

Do you ever feel that someone is touching you, but when you look there is nobody there?)
(Have you noticed that food or drink seems to have an unusual taste recently?)

RATE OTHER HALLUCINATIONS AND DELUSIONAL
ELABORATION: *Exclude hypochondriacal and nihilistic delusions
rated in (90) and (91).*   (70)

   1 = Sensation of touch, food tastes burnt, etc., but subject puzzled by the
      experience. No delusional elaboration.

   2 = Delusional elaboration in addition, e.g. fantasy lover, food poisoned, etc.

Project no.

1 2

Subject no.

3 4 5

Card no.

6 7

8 9 10

15. DELUSIONS

Definition

Delusions may be of two kinds, primary and secondary. Both kinds are rated together in the following symptoms except where specified. For example, primary delusions are specifically rated in symptom (82). They are defined here for convenience.

Primary delusions are based upon experiences in which a subject suddenly becomes convinced that a particular set of events has a special meaning (e.g. a subject undergoing a liver biopsy suddenly felt he had been chosen by God). The delusion cannot be explained and it is not shared by other members of the subject's cultural or social group.

Secondary delusions are delusional elaborations of primary delusions or other basic phenomena such as derealisation, depersonalisation, perceptual distortions, hallucinations, thought echo, mood changes, etc.

Above cut-off questions, likely to elicit delusions if present, are included in many of the preceding sections. There may also be evidence in the case-record or in the subject's spontaneous account.

IF NO EVIDENCE AT ALL THAT DELUSIONS ARE PRESENT, CUT OFF → SECTION 16.

RECORD IF ANY PSYCHOTIC PHENOMENA PRESENT, OTHER THAN DELUSIONS, USE JUDGEMENT AS TO WHETHER TO PROCEED BEYOND CUT-OFF.

Cut off

IF ANY EVIDENCE FOR DELUSIONS, ASK ALL QUESTIONS NOT IN BRACKETS, AND ANY FURTHER QUESTIONS WHICH SEEM INDICATED.

RATING OF PARTIAL AND FULL DELUSIONS.

In general, all delusions are rated as follows:

    1 = Partial delusions, which are expressed with doubt, or as possibilities which the subject entertains but is not certain about. This rating should not be used if it is clear that full delusions have been present during the month, or if the subject has acted as if fully deluded.

    2 = Full delusions have been present at some time during the month. Fully convinced. No insight.

A useful question to elucidate the difference between partial and full delusions is as follows:

Even when you seem to be most convinced, do you really feel in the back of your mind that it might well not be true, that it might be imagination?

15A. DELUSIONS OF CONTROL

Definition
The subject's will is replaced by that of some external agency. A simple statement that the radio is controlling the subject is not sufficient. (This statement, alone, should be rated 8.) The subject must describe a replacement of will by some other force.
    Do not include feeling that life is planned and directed by fate, or that the future is present already in embryo, or that subject is not very strong-willed, or that voices give subject orders. Do not include simple identification with God or being under God's direction. Do not include subcultural or hysterical possession states or multiple personality (→ 100).

Do you feel under the control of some force or power other than yourself?
(As though you were a robot or a zombie without a will of your own?)
(As though you were possessed by someone or something else?)
(What is that like?)
(Does this force make your movements for you without your willing it, or use your voice, or your handwriting? Does it replace your personality? What is the explanation?)

    ☐ (71)

RATE DELUSIONS OF CONTROL.
    1 = Partial delusions   2 = Full delusions

15B. MISINTERPRETATIONS, MISIDENTIFICATION AND DELUSIONS OF REFERENCE

Definition
Delusions of reference: Do not include simple self-consciousness or feeling that subject attracts comment, even if critical. These are rated under symptom 31.

There must be elaboration: e.g. someone crosses his knees in order to indicate that the subject is homosexual; or the whole neighbourhood is gossiping.

Delusional misinterpretations, etc. This is an extension of the delusion of reference, so that not only do people seem to refer to subject, but situations appear to be deliberately created to test him (exclude situations of medical treatment), or objects appear to have special meanings.

Do people seem to drop hints about you or say things with a double meaning, or do things in a special way so as to convey a meaning?
Does everyone seem to gossip about you?
(Do people follow you about or check up on you or record your movements?)
(How do they do it? Why?)
(Are there people about who are not what they seem to be?)
RATE DELUSIONS OF REFERENCE.

☐ (72)

    1 = Partial delusions   2 = Full delusions.

Do things seem to be specially arranged?
(Is an experiment going on, to test you out?)
(Do you see any reference to yourself on TV or in the papers?)
(Do you ever seem to see special meanings in advertisements, or shop windows, or in the way things are arranged?)
(How do you explain this?)
RATE DELUSIONAL MISINTERPRETATION AND
MISIDENTIFICATION.

☐ (73)

    1 = Partial delusions   2 = Full delusions

15C. DELUSIONS OF PERSECUTION

Is anyone deliberately trying to harm you, e.g. trying to poison you or kill you?
(How? Is there an organisation like the Mafia behind it?)
(Is there any other kind of persecution? How do you explain this?)
RATE DELUSIONS OF PERSECUTION.

☐ (74)

    1 = Partial delusions   2 = Full delusions

15D. EXPANSIVE DELUSIONS

Do you think that people are organising things specially to help you?

RATE DELUSIONS OF ASSISTANCE.

☐ (75)

    1 = Partial delusions   2 = Full delusions

Is there anything special about you? Do you have special abilities or powers?
(Can you read people's thoughts?)
(Is there a special purpose or mission to your life?)
(Are you especially clever or inventive? How do you explain this?)
RATE DELUSIONS OF GRANDIOSE ABILITIES.

☐ (76)

    1 = Partial delusions   2 = Full delusions

(Are you a very prominent person or related to someone prominent, like Royalty?)
(Are you very rich or famous?)
(How do you explain this?)
RATE DELUSIONS OF GRANDIOSE IDENTITY: *(Exclude religious identification.)*

☐ (77)

   1 = Partial delusions   2 = Full delusions

15E. DELUSIONS CONCERNING VARIOUS TYPES OF INFLUENCE AND PRIMARY DELUSIONS

Are you a very religious person?
(Specially close to Christ or God?)
(Can God communicate with you? How?)
(Are you yourself a saint?)
(How do you explain this?)
RATE RELIGIOUS DELUSIONS: *Including delusional religious explanations of other experiences. Exclude intense religious belief or purely subcultural beliefs.*

☐ (78)

   1 = Partial delusions   2 = Full delusions

How do you explain the things that have been happening? (SPECIFY)
Is there anything like hypnotism, telepathy, or the occult going on?
What is the explanation?
INCLUDE DELUSIONAL EXPLANATIONS IN TERMS OF PARANORMAL PHENOMENA: *e.g. hypnotism, telepathy, magic, witchcraft, etc. Exclude purely subcultural beliefs,* → *83.*

☐ (79)

  .1 = Partial delusions   2 = Full delusions

Is anything like electricity, or X-rays, or radio-waves affecting you?
(In what way? What is the explanation?)
INCLUDE DELUSIONAL EXPLANATIONS IN TERMS OF PHYSICAL FORCES: *e.g. radio, television, X-rays, electricity, transmitters, microphones, machines of various kinds.*

☐ (80)

   1 = Partial delusions   2 = Full delusions

DELUSIONS OF ALIEN FORCES PENETRATING OR CONTROLLING MIND (OR BODY).

☐ (81)

Include any delusion, whether rated elsewhere or not, which involves an external force penetrating the subject's mind or body, e.g. rays turn liver to gold, alien thoughts pierce skull or are inserted into mind, hypnotism makes patient levitate, a spirit speaks with subject's voice, a radio transmitter has been implanted into brain and broadcasts thoughts or controls actions, etc.

   1 = Partial delusions   2 = Full delusions

Choose a likely delusion, and ask:

How did it come into your mind that this was the explanation?
(Did it happen suddenly? How did it begin?)

RATE PRIMARY DELUSIONS: *Based upon experiences in which subject suddenly becomes convinced that a particular set of events has a special meaning. (See definition on page 214.) Not based on mood or explanation of other abnormal experiences.*

(82)

    1 = Partial delusions   2 = Full delusions

15F. OTHER DELUSIONS

(Examiner should question as appropriate.)

RATE SUBCULTURALLY INFLUENCED DELUSIONS: *Include only subjects who belong to small groups with definitely idiosyncratic beliefs; small sects, tribes, 'secret societies', etc.*

(83)

    0 = No significant subcultural influence. For example, an English subject believing he is influenced by TV would be rated (0) since, although the delusion depends on TV being available in England, it is not in any way specific to a small subcultural group.

    1 = One or more of the 'delusions' rated earlier could easily be no more than a belief shared by other members of the subject's subcultural group, e.g. the Pentecostal church with the gift of tongues. Voodoo, witchcraft, communicating with God, are other examples of beliefs which may be taken quite literally by groups of people who are not clinically deluded. Rate (1) if subject holds such beliefs without elaborating them further.

    2 = As (1), but because of excitement, expansiveness, depression, confusion, intellectual retardation, etc., the subject holds the beliefs with exceptional fervour and conviction, or elaborates them further. Such a subject might well be regarded as abnormal by other members of his own sect or group.

    3 = More specific delusional states, e.g. Koro, Witigo, etc.

(Do you have any reason to be jealous of anybody?)

MORBID JEALOUSY.

(84)

    1 = Partial delusions   2 = Full delusions

DELUSION OF PREGNANCY.

(85)

    1 = Partial delusions   2 = Full delusions

SEXUAL DELUSIONS: *Any delusion with sexual content, e.g. fantasy lover, sex changing, etc. Do not include an untrue claim that a subject is married or has children.*

(86)

    1 = Partial delusions   2 = Full delusions

Have you had any unusual experience or adventures recently?

RATE FANTASTIC DELUSIONS, DELUSIONAL MEMORIES,
DELUSIONAL CONFABULATIONS, FANTASTIC DELUSIONS:
Confabulation: Subject makes up delusions on the spot. Very rare.
Delusional memories: Subject seems to be describing actual memories.
Describes the same delusions time and again. Not confabulations.
Rare, e.g. 'I came down to earth on a silver star.' Fantastic delusions: (87)
The commonest of the three, e.g. England's coast melting.

1 = Partial delusions   2 = Full delusions

15G. SIMPLE DELUSIONS BASED ON GUILT,
    DEPERSONALISATION, HYPOCHONDRIASIS, ETC.

Definition

These symptoms often appear to be based on a depressed mood and are relatively
consistent and unelaborated. Do not include more bizarre elaborations of any of
them, e.g. having a metal nose = symptom 87, not 89. Having been turned into
another specified person = possibly symptom 71, not 90. Liver turned to lead by
X-rays = symptoms 80 and 81, not 91. England's coast melting = symptom 87,
not 92.

Do you feel you have committed a crime, or sinned greatly, or deserve punishment?
(Have you felt that your presence might contaminate or ruin other
people?) (88)
RATE DELUSIONS OF GUILT.
  1 = Subject has brought ruin to family by being in present condition, or thinks
      that symptoms are a punishment for not doing better, etc. Does not
      elaborate as in (2).
  2 = Subject says has sinned greatly or committed some terrible crime or brought
      ruin upon the world. May feel deserving of punishment, even of death or
      hell-fire, because of it.

(Do you think your appearance is normal?)
RATE SIMPLE DELUSIONS CONCERNING APPEARANCE: (89)
(Nose too large, teeth misshapen, body crooked, etc.)
  1 = Strong feeling that there is something wrong with appearance; subject looks
      old or ugly or dead, skin cracked, teeth misshapen, nose too large, body
      crooked, etc. Can be reassured temporarily. There may be only one limited
      preoccupation.
  2 = Subject acts accordingly (plastic operations, etc.)

(Is anything the matter with your brain?)
RATE DELUSIONS OF DEPERSONALISATION: *Subject has no* (90)
head, does not exist, hollow instead of a brain, etc.
  1 = Unable to think, no thoughts in head, feels *as though* he has no brain or as
      though it does not function at all.
  2 = Symptom more intense. Subject has no head, no brain, does not exist.

(Is anything the matter with your body?)

RATE HYPOCHONDRIACAL DELUSIONS: *Subject has incurable cancer, bowels are stopped up, insides are rotting, etc.*

(91)

  1 = Subject feels body is unhealthy, rotten, diseased, but without the force of (2).
  2 = Subject has incurable cancer, bowels are stopped up or rotting away, etc.

(Do you have the feeling that something terrible is going to happen? What?)

RATE DELUSIONS OF CATASTROPHE: *World is about to end, some catastrophe has happened or will occur, everything is evil and will be destroyed.*

(92)

  1 = Subject feels sense of impending doom; something awful will happen. Non-specific but out of proportion to circumstances.
  2 = Delusional conviction that world is about to end or some other enormous catastrophe is about to occur or has occurred. World is dirty, decayed, rotten: i.e. further delusional elaboration of (1).

15H. GENERAL RATINGS OF DELUSIONS AND HALLUCINATIONS

(Include both partial and full delusions.)

CONSIDER BOTH DELUSIONS AND HALLUCINATIONS IN FOLLOWING RATINGS.

RATE SYSTEMATISATION OF DELUSIONS.

(93)

Scoring:
  0 = No delusions or hallucinations.
  1 = Delusions and hallucinations not elaborated into a general system affecting much of the subject's experience. Include encapsulated delusions or isolated hallucinations.
  2 = Some systematic elaboration, but substantial areas of the subject's experiences are not affected.
  3 = Subject interprets practically all his experience in delusional terms.

RATE EVASIVENESS.

(94)

Scoring:
  0 = No attempt at concealment suspected.
  1 = Examiner suspects that there may be (either) delusions or hallucinations in the background, but the subject is not concealing much of the psychopathology.
  2 = Examiner suspects that there is a considerable preoccupation with delusions (even a delusional system) or hallucinations, but the subject tries to conceal them.
  3 = No concealment but other delusions or hallucinations probably present. Not elicited because of poor intelligence and education or incoherence or muteness, etc.

OVERALL RATING OF PREOCCUPATION WITH DELUSIONS
AND HALLUCINATIONS.

□ (95)

Scoring:
- 0 = No delusions or hallucinations.
- 1 = No delusions or hallucinations definitely rated but examiner suspects that they may be present.
- 2 = Preoccupied with past delusions or hallucinations only. Not actively deluded or hallucinated at present.
- 3 = Delusions or hallucinations definitely present but subject is not preoccupied with them for much of the time. Can turn attention to other things without difficulty.
- 4 = Delusions or hallucinations present and take up most of the subject's attention. Preoccupied to the exclusion of many other matters.
- 5 = Patient can hardly discuss anything but delusions.

RATE ACTING OUT DELUSIONS
(Rate from case-record, etc.)

□ (96)

Scoring:
- 0 = No delusions or hallucinations.
- 1 = Subject able to keep delusions or hallucinations to himself, or to confide them only to a few trusted people (sympathetic relatives, friends, doctors, etc.). He does not express them in public nor act upon them. Does not talk out loud to voices.
- 2 = Subject has acted upon delusions or hallucinations during past month, or expressed them in public (i.e. outside the small circle of people who would be expected to be sympathetic). This has not, however, resulted in severe social disturbance or a social crisis.
- 3 = As (2) but acting out, or public expression, has resulted in severe social disturbance or a social crisis.

16. SENSORIUM AND FACTORS AFFECTING

** Have you had any lapses of memory recently?
(Have there been any periods in which you completely forgot what happened?)
(What was it like?)
(How do you explain it?)

RATE FUGUES, BLACKOUTS, AMNESIA LASTING MORE
THAN ONE HOUR: *irrespective of aetiology.*

□ (97)

- 1 = less than 12 hours.
- 2 = 12–24 hours.
- 3 = more than 24 hours.

** What medicines or drugs do you take?
(Do you take anything for your nerves or your mood?)
(Obtain list of drugs.)
(Who prescribes?)

RATE DRUG ABUSE DURING MONTH. *One category only.* □ (98)
    1 = Cannabis.
    2 = Amytal, etc.
    3 = LSD, amphetamine, etc.
    4 = Cocaine, heroin, etc.

** May I ask about your drinking habits? How much do you usually drink each day?
(Is alcohol in any way a problem for you? In what way?)

(CHECK LIST: *Present on card if needed.* During the past month have you:
had family problems because of drinking?
missed work because of drinking?
had morning shakes or other withdrawal symptoms?
had blackouts for several hours?
heard voices or seen visions?)

RATE ALCOHOL ABUSE DURING PAST MONTH. □ (99)
    1 = Agrees alcohol has been a problem but not 2.
    2 = Any check-list item applies.

RATE DISSOCIATIVE STATES DURING PAST MONTH:
*'Narrowing of consciousness which serves an unconscious purpose and
is commonly accompanied or followed by a selective amnesia',
e.g. trance, possession state, fugue, hypersomnia, stupor, etc.
Do not include if caused by drugs, alcohol, epilepsy, etc.* □ (100)
    1 = Present during the past month, but not at examination.
    2 = Present at examination.

RATE CONVERSION SYMPTOMS, *e.g. paralysis, anaesthesia,
blindness, tremor, seizures, etc. if mentioned during interview.* □ (101)
    1 = Present during month, not at examination.
    2 = Present at examination.

RATE CLOUDING OR STUPOR AT
EXAMINATION □ (102)
    1 = Clouding: Inadequate comprehension of external impressions, with per-
        plexity, and impairment of attention and orientation.
    2 = Stupor: Subject appears comatose but there is no clouding or impairment
        of consciousness.

IF ANY SUSPICION OF POOR MEMORY OR DISORIENTATION:

May I ask one or two standard questions we ask of everybody?
How old are you?
Can you tell me the year and the month?
What is the name of the Prime Minister?

RATE ORGANIC IMPAIRMENT OF MEMORY. *See glossary for definition.*   ☐ (103)

   1 = Mild.
   2 = Moderate.
   3 = Severe.

17. INSIGHT

** Do you think there is anything the matter with you?
   (What do you think it is?)
   (Could it be a nervous condition?)
   (What do you think the cause is?)
   (Why did you need to come to hospital?)
   (Do you think (*specify delusions or hallucinations*) were part of a nervous condition?)

IF PSYCHOTIC SYMPTOMS (i.e. SYMPTOMS FROM SECTIONS 12–15):   ☐ (104)

   0 = Full insight (in intelligent subject, able to appreciate the issues involved).
   1 = As much insight into the nature of the condition as social background and intelligence allow.
   2 = Agrees to a nervous condition but examiner feels that subject does not really accept the explanation in terms of a nervous illness (e.g. gives delusional explanation, the result of persecution, or rays, etc.).
   3 = Denies nervous condition entirely.
   9 = Psychotic illness not present.

IF NEUROTIC SYMPTOMS (i.e. SYMPTOMS FROM SECTIONS 1–11 ONLY):   ☐ (105)

   0 = Full insight (in intelligent subject, able to appreciate the issues involved).
   1 = As much insight into the nature of the condition as social background and intelligence allow.
   2 = Gives physical explanation for neurotic symptoms.
   3 = Denies neurotic symptoms entirely.
   9 = Neurotic illness not present.

** Of all the problems you have told me about, which one affects you most?
   How much does it interfere with your work or your relationships with other people?
   (Have you actually been out of work, or been unable to do the housework, or go shopping, travelling, etc., during the past month?)
   (Have the symptoms impaired your efficiency in any other way?)

RATE SOCIAL IMPAIRMENT DUE TO NEUROTIC CONDITION.   ☐ (106)

   0 = No neurotic or psychotic symptoms present.
   1 = Neurotic symptoms present but little diminution of subject's efficiency or interference with everyday activities.

2 = Neurotic symptoms interfere with subject's efficiency to a moderate extent but are not incapacitating, e.g. subject neglects housework or can't enjoy leisure activities or social relationships, or finds work-efficiency reduced because of worry, tension, irritability, depression, anxiety, etc. Subject does not, however, stop work altogether or completely neglect household.

3 = Subject severely incapacitated by neurotic symptoms: had to have at least a week off work during past month; was housebound for a week or more; was actively withdrawn from all social relationships, etc. The subject does not have to be totally incapacitated for the whole month for this rating to be made, but impairment has to be very severe.

8 = Examiner unsure.

9 = Psychotic condition present.

(If both psychotic and neurotic condition, rate whichever shows more impairment.)

RATE SOCIAL IMPAIRMENT DUE TO PSYCHOTIC CONDITION

(10?

0 = No neurotic or psychotic symptoms present.

1 = Psychotic symptoms present but little diminution of subject's efficiency or interference with everyday activities.

2 = Psychotic symptoms interfere with subject's efficiency to a moderate extent but are not incapacitating, e.g. subject neglects housework or can't enjoy leisure activities or social relationships, or finds work-efficiency reduced. Subject does not, however, stop work altogether or completely neglect household.

3 = Subject severely incapacitated by psychotic symptoms: had to have at least a week off work during past month; was housebound for a week or more; was actively withdrawn from all social relationships, etc. The subject does not have to be totally incapacitated for the whole month for this rating to be made, but impairment has to be very severe.

8 = Examiner unsure.

9 = Neurotic condition, and no psychotic condition, present.

FINAL QUESTION

** Have there been any other things lately that I haven't covered?
Specify:

Note here any points that seem to be important or unusual about the subject or the interview which are not covered in the schedule.

Reconsider schedule to make sure that all obligatory questions have been asked. Also consider whether behaviour, affect and speech ratings can be made or whether further observation or examination is necessary. IF NOT, THIS IS THE END OF THE INTERVIEW.

18–20. BEHAVIOUR, AFFECT AND SPEECH

RATINGS

    0 = Symptom absent.
    1 = Present in fairly severe degree, or very severe but intermittent during.
       interview.
    2 = Present in very severe degree and almost continuous during interview.
    8 = Examiner not sure.
    9 = Subject not examined, or examination not appropriate.

N.B. If in doubt, rate (0). A rating of (1) means there is no doubt about the symptom being present in fairly severe form.

Behaviour during interview

Self-neglect (cleanliness, shaven, make-up, state of hair and clothes).   (108)

Bizarre appearance (secret documents openly displayed, special clothes or ornaments with symbolic significance, etc. Do not include mannerisms or posturing = symptom 116).   (109)

Slowness and underactivity (sits abnormally still, walks abnormally slowly, delay in performing movements).   (110)

Agitation (fidgety, restlessness, pacing, frequent unnecessary movements).   (111)

Gross excitement and violence (throws things, runs or jumps about, waves arms wildly, shouts or screams).   (112)

Irreverent behaviour (sings, facetious, silly jokes, flippant remarks, unduly familiar).   (113)

Distractibility (stops talking or changes subject due to distraction by trivial noises or events outside the room or turns attention to furniture, etc.).   (114)

Embarrassing behaviour (making sexual suggestions or advances to interviewer; loss of social restraint – scratches genitals, passes loud flatus, etc.).   (115)

Mannerisms and posturing (odd, stylised movements or acts, usually idiosyncratic to the patient, often suggestive of special meaning or purpose: assuming and maintaining uncomfortable or inappropriate postures).   (116)

Stereotypies, etc. (constant repetition of movements or postures such as rocking, rubbing, nodding, grimacing: no special significance).   (117)

Behaves as if hallucinated (non-verbal: as though hears voices or visions: lips move soundlessly, looks round, giggles to self – not just from embarrassment, shyness, etc.).   (118)

Catatonic movements
(Negativism: does the opposite of what he is asked.
Ambitendence: begins to take proffered hand, then withdraws; etc.
Echopraxia: imitates examiner's movement.
Flexibilitas cerea: arm remains where it is put, for at least 15 seconds.
Mitgehen: excessive co-operation in passive movement.
Echolalia: imitates words and phrases with same intonation and inflection of voice.)
(These items can be separately rated in special projects.)

□ (119)

Affect during interview
Observed anxiety (tense worried look or posture, fearful apprehensive look, frightened tone of voice, tremor).

□ (120)

Observed depression (sad, mournful look, tears, gloomy tone of
voice, deep sighing, voice chokes on distressing topic).

□ (121)

Histrionic (feelings expressed in exaggerated, dramatic, histrionic
manner).

□ (122)

Hypomanic affect (unduly cheerful, smiling, euphoric,
elated).

□ (123)

Hostile irritability (unco-operative, irritable, angry, overtly hostile,
discontented, haughty, antagonistic).

□ (124)

Suspicion.

□ (125)

Perplexity (puzzlement).

□ (126)

Lability of mood (whether lability of one mood, or changing from
one mood to another).

□ (127)

Blunted affect (expressionless face and voice, uniform blunting
whatever the topic of conversation, indifference to distressing
topics, whether delusional or normal).

□ (128)

   1 = Blunting not uniform, e.g. at times responds affectively but
      at other times is markedly flat; or responds with some
      evidence of affect, but definitely less than expected.
   2 = Severe and uniform blunting.

Incongruity of affect (emotion is shown, but not congruent
with topic).

□ (129)

Speech during interview
Slow speech (long pauses before answering, long pauses between
words).

□ (130)

Pressure of speech (more copious speech than normal, too rapid
speech, very loud voice, too circumstantial speech).

□ (131)

Non-social speech (talks, mutters, whispers out loud, out of
context of conversation with examiner).

□ (132)

Muteness
 1 = Almost mute, fewer than twenty words in all.
 2 = Totally mute.

☐ (133)

Restricted quantity of speech (subject frequently fails to answer, questions have to be repeated, restricted to minimum necessary, no extra sentences, no additional comments).

☐ (134)

Neologisms and idosyncratic use of words or phrases, e.g. 'One is called "Per-God" and the other is called "Per-the-Devil"', '... miracle-willed through God's "tarn-harn"...', 'Well, there is a frequenting of clairvoyance...': 'Per-God', 'Per-the-Devil' and 'tarn-harn' are neologisms; 'frequenting of clairvoyance' is an example of ordinary words used idiosyncratically. DO NOT RATE THIS SYMPTOM PRESENT UNLESS EXAMPLES ARE WRITTEN DOWN.

☐ (135)

Disorder of content of speech
Three types of disordered content are specified: in each case, the effect is to make it very difficult to grasp what the subject means. However, the symptoms are defined in terms of specific components so that it should, in most cases, be possible to say whether one, two, or all three symptoms are present. If in doubt, rate hierarchically, i.e. rate incoherence in preference to flight of ideas and flight of ideas in preference to poverty of speech.
 If the patient does not talk enough to give a rateable sample of speech, rate all three symptoms Y.

Incoherence of speech. The subject's meaning is obscured by dis-torted grammar, lack of logical connection between one part of a sentence and another or between sentences, sudden irrelevances or 'Knight's move', grossly pedantic phrases, answering off the point, etc. For example:

☐ (136)

 'We've seen the downfall of the radium crown by the Roman Catholics, whereas when you come to see the drinking side of the business, God saw that Noah, if he lost his reason, he got nobody there to look after them.'
 'I did suggest to you, that intrinsic or congenital sentiment or refinement of disposition would be so miracle-willed through God's "tarn-harn" as to assume quite the opposite.'
 'I believe we live in a world, in an age, where the elements are a force that elders of professionalism hope, not to conquer, but to control.'
 'What's your address?' 'It's supposed to be Salisbury near Birmingham.'
(*Vorbeireden.*)
DO NOT RATE THIS SYMPTOM PRESENT UNLESS EXAMPLES ARE WRITTEN DOWN.
A rating of 2 means that very little normal speech is present.
N.B. A free flow of delusions is not necessarily incoherent. A subject may talk about delusions quite coherently.

Flight of ideas. Words are associated together inappropriately by sound or rhyme (clang association). Although the original aim of the sentence may quickly be lost, a path can be traced through associations of the white–black–coffin or ring–wrong variety, or through associations with distracting stimuli, e.g.

☐ (137)

'How is your appetite?' 'I feel as if I have lost my appetite. I have had an orange. A real juicy orange.' (Sees patient walking past window.) 'She is going for E.C.T. Etcetera treatment or teddy bear's picnic. I call it.'

DO NOT RATE THIS SYMPTOM PRESENT UNLESS EXAMPLES ARE WRITTEN DOWN.

A rating of 2 means that very little normal speech is present.

Poverty of content of speech. The subject talks freely but so vaguely that little information is given in spite of the number of words used: rambles on without coming to a point; may wander far from original theme. Exclude incoherence or flight of ideas. Rate only if severe and always give written example.

☐ (138)

Misleading answers. Subject's answers are misleading because answers 'yes' or 'no' to everything, or frequent self-contradictions, or appears to be deliberately misleading. Do not include incoherence, flight of ideas or poverty of speech here.

☐ (139)

Re-rate adequacy of interview

☐ (140)

    0 = Ratings made adequately represent the symptoms present.
    1 = Some problem but key symptoms have been rated.
    2 = Serious question as to adequacy of interview for rating key
        symptoms (other than sections 18–20).
    3 = *Only* sections 18–20 could be rated.

Check that every box has an entry except those below ticked cut-off points.

Complete coding sheet if one is being used.

SYMPTOM INDEX

Page references are given for the glossary definitions and the PSE.

SUBJECT INDEX

NAME INDEX

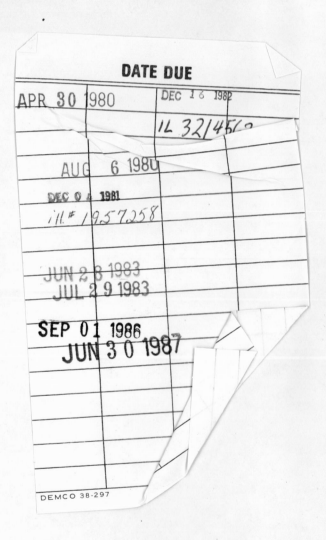